Fix Yo
High Blood Pressure
in 90 Days or Less

.

Fix Your
High Blood Pressure
in 90 Days or Less

Scientific Methods to Break Free from Life Long Prescription Meds

Dr Joseph Amagada FRCOG, MBSLM

FIRST EDITION JULY 2022

Book design by Publishing Push

ISBNs:
Paperback: 978-1-80227-558-2
eBook: 978-1-80227-559-9

Subscribe to receive weekly emails from Dr Joe
Visit: drjoeconnect.com to subscribe
Blog: thedrjoe.com

This book is dedicated to my three children – Renée, Wesley and Bradley for missing out on "Daddy time". Daddy spent a disproportionate amount of time in the hospital working during your growing up years, so this one is for you.

Table of Contents

Preface

My decision to write this book was based entirely on my wish to share what I know and what my personal experience has been with managing high blood pressure with the rest of the world and, of course, the hypertension community more specifically. I decided some years ago to take a different approach to dealing with my hypertension problems. It was a rocky journey at first because I had no road map to follow.

The fact I am a physician made no difference at all in the beginning of my journey. I was blazing a trail devoid of any structural format whatsoever. I wished at the time that there was a proven path I could simply leap into and follow all the way through. None existed. At least not one that had a structure along with scientific backing anyway. If, like me, you needed an evidence-based approach, then the onus was on you to do some digging yourself and that's what I did.

I can confirm it wasn't fun at all because I spent months of intense research dissecting all there was to know in medical literature and working out how to apply it to my everyday management of high blood pressure. It was hard toil, but it paid off because those thousands of hours with my neck deep into research and testing what works and what doesn't, has made me a better physician, a more integrative medical doctor and a lifestyle medical expert, and you are going to be the beneficiary of my newfound love of lifestyle medicine. This book ensures you don't go through that level of toil like I did. What a relief that must be for you.

What do doctors do for high blood pressure? We provide prescriptions for patients after some initial tests to find a cause. Lifestyle modification is usually given a lip service, therefore not taken seriously and that's a mistake as I have come to realise on my journey. Yes, prescription medications do have a role but too many people are needlessly on prescription pills for far too long, mainly because it is seen as the only way out. Worse is the fact that prescription medications only successfully control hypertension in 35% of users. What about the other 65% who struggle?

I did belong to that 65% and it was reflected in my kidney function as it was going downhill as the years went by. Until I decided to take this path of seeking lifestyle medicine. I succeeded in controlling my blood pressure naturally, but could I help others do the same? It turns out I could.

One of the first things I did after writing this book was present the manuscript to two medical doctors whose work I admire very much. They have been in the business of incorporating lifestyle medicine into their medical practice longer than I have, so their opinion on the content of this book was particularly important to me. The first physician to go over the manuscript is a popular doctor in the United States. He has been around for decades preaching the gospel of lifestyle medicine on his website, his clinics, on social media and gives talks all over the world. I know it is a cliché, but you could argue he has seen it all having been around the world of medicine for this long. He should know a good self-help health book when he sees one. His name is Dr Michael Klaper, MD – one of America's most loved physicians. I wanted his take on what I had written here. Guess what? Dr Klaper liked it. He liked it because the book is simply a well-researched and well-presented helpful resource. Here is what Dr Klaper had to say:

> "I never expected a book on high blood pressure to be a great read, but what a pleasant surprise – and valuable resource – Dr Joseph Amagada has given to us all. In *Fix Your High Blood Pressure in 90 Days or Less*, Dr Joseph Amagada explores and explains the mechanisms of this common and life-threatening disorder with crisp explanations, colourful examples, and even historical vignettes. An experienced physician and an entertaining writer who clearly loves to teach, Dr Amagada makes clear why blood pressure goes up, how to measure it accurately, and, most importantly, how to keep blood pressures in a healthy range with diet and lifestyle practices that will benefit every aspect of your life.
>
> After reading *Fix Your High Blood Pressure in 90 Days or Less*, most lay people will know as much or more about elevated blood pressure than their doctor does, and most physicians will be far better able to effectively treat their patients with hypertension. I will recommend this book to my patients and colleagues, and no doubt will even employ some of his sage wisdom in my own life."
>
> Michael Klaper, MD
> Physician and author

The second physician who was kind enough to read the manuscript and offer his opinion was Dr Joel Kahn. Dr Kahn is a Cardiologist who runs the Kahn Center for Cardiac Longevity in Michigan and also a Clinical Professor at the Wayne State University of Medicine also in Michigan. Dr Kahn sees hypertension patients every working day of his life, so he should know what a good high blood pressure book is. Here's what Dr Kahn said about this book:

> "Blood pressure control dominates my integrative cardiology practice. I spend more time on home blood pressure monitoring than any other home habit. Joseph Amagada, MD, has written a guide to fixing high blood pressure with as natural techniques as possible. I will have my patients study this bible of blood pressure knowledge and they will benefit from it. Two thumbs up"
>
> Joel Kahn, MD, FACC
> Author, #1 sellers: The Whole Heart Solution, Dead Execs, The Plant Based Solution

I have been spreading the message in this book on various platforms and most of my students have successfully brought their blood pressures right down to where it belongs. I do not want testimonials to take up too much space in this book, but sharing one or two with you wouldn't be a bad idea, would it? How about these ones:

> "Dr Joe is an excellent teacher because he not only talks the talk, but he also walks the walk. He demonstrates clear and practical solutions to our health issues with great dietary guidelines, suggestions and demonstrations of lifestyle changes to improve ourselves. This has resulted in me losing 30 lbs and achieving an average blood pressure of 120/70. Also, his teaching has guided me from a pre-diabetic A1C blood glucose level to normal readings. I am deeply grateful to Dr Joe. I highly recommend his lifestyle modifications to fix your high blood pressure and I'm looking forward to reading his

book and giving it to my friends and family for their edification."

Ellen Ogiri – Florida, USA

"I have had a clean bill of health for a long time till I got pregnant. In my third trimester, I started having issues with high blood pressure. This continued after birth when I was put on various blood pressure medications. In my search for understanding and solutions, I stumbled upon a YouTube video of a man demonstrating a set of exercises he boldly claimed could help you beat high blood pressure: the ultimate nitric oxide dump exercise. His name was Dr Joe and he had convincing videos on combating high blood pressure. It was intriguing; new insight and a different approach to the use of exercises and healthy eating primarily in nipping high blood pressure in the bud. His advice on sets of exercises, recipes and other lifestyle changes are borne out of practical application in his own life. With Dr Joe, he tries everything on himself and, therefore, can vouch and speak to its effectiveness. A few months after meeting Dr Joe, my doctor took me off all my medications and it's been a year and a half and still counting. All thanks to this humble, selfless and dedicated man, I have stopped using medications and have stayed with his prescribed exercises, diet and variety of teas leading to my blood pressure being within normal range."

Cindy Garbrah – East Midlands, United Kingdom

"Hi Dr Joe. I have been on the nitric oxide dump for about two months now. I started at 5 reps for each exercise and am now on 20 reps twice a day. I also walk about 45 minutes daily plus eat about 6 servings of greens and fruits per day. I was going to start with the teas and turmeric, but I got scared. The reason is my BP readings as outlined below for the last ten days: 105/65, 120/67, 111/68, 116/70, 116/70, 125/71, 121/76, 115/72, 115/73, 115/68. Imagine what will happen to those readings when I start the teas and turmeric. Your interventions work big time, Dr Joe. Thank you ever so much for what you are doing for us. If anyone was a doubting Thomas, doubt no more."

Tulani Sithole – South Africa

I have coached, and still coach, over a thousand people from all four corners of the earth to overcome this high blood pressure disease. If you are someone who listens to clean advice and can follow through with simple instructions, you will see a difference in your blood pressure readings. That's a promise. And, with a little bit more effort, your doctor may just say those words you've been waiting to hear regarding your lifelong dependency on prescription pills: "Time to come off those medications now." Fantastic news!

Will it be you receiving the good news next? Read on...

Introduction

Hypertension, for avoidance of doubt, is known in plain English as high blood pressure. So, for the purpose of this book, the terms "hypertension" and "high blood pressure" will be used interchangeably.

High blood pressure is a scourge. It ruins lives. It unsettles families by either incapacitating one or more members of a family or just shortening the life expectancy of a family member. High blood pressure, like any other devastating disease, is never good news. But the march of high blood pressure to destroy lives and make people feel unhappy and miserable can be stopped. And that's my aim in this book. I want to bring to you, in simple plain English, the education you need to understand this disease from the bottom up in scores of pages that you should enjoy reading. This book has been written in a very practical way as I bring my own personal experience of managing the disease in myself into play. So, you will read about my personal anecdotes in this book which should help you understand the disease a lot more on a personal level. That's a promise I intend to keep and will keep in the entire length and breadth of this book.

How bad is high blood pressure as a global problem? The prevalence of high blood pressure has been on the rise relentlessly in the last thirty years especially in the age group 30–79.

This upward swing in prevalence is ahead of type 2 diabetes. Hypertension and type 2 diabetes share a lot in common beyond the "popularity" stakes.

Both conditions commonly coexist in the same individual than could be explained by chance alone. In fact, hypertension is twice as common in individuals with diabetes than those without. In the US, hypertension coexists in 30% of type 1 diabetes patients but is found in 50–80% of those with type 2 diabetes. That high occurrence in type 2 diabetes tells us there is a common string in the origin of both conditions. That relationship will be explored in the later chapters of this book.

A detailed study conducted by a network of physicians and researchers spanning the period between 1990 and 2019, has revealed hypertension now affects 1.28 billion people globally[1]. This is in the age group 30–79. Sadly, close to 50% of these affected individuals do not even know they have the condition. The study covered 184 countries. The study, therefore, represents the most comprehensive analysis of the current trend of hypertension ever carried out. With the world population at the time of writing being 7.8 billion, that is a huge chunk of people harbouring the prospect of potential complications of high blood pressure if poorly managed.

In the UK, 11.8 million people in the age group 16 years and over have high blood pressure in England alone[2]. That is 26.2% of England's adult population. The picture in the US is worse. Nearly half of US adults have hypertension[3]. We are talking 108 million people in that western part of the world. The Center for Disease Control and Prevention data for 2018 suggests hypertension contributed directly or indirectly to nearly half a million deaths[4]. This high prevalence of high blood pressure and the associated complications can be traced to the way our lifestyles have evolved in this twenty-first century. We can blame fast-moving lifestyles that are arguably unhealthy. And with those fast-moving lifestyles spreading globally like wildfire, it is not surprising hypertension is becoming a scourge. But I do not want to get into that just yet. Let us save that for later.

In today's world, non-communicable diseases have become dominant unlike centuries ago when communicable diseases were rife. High blood pressure is certainly high on that list of non-communicable diseases.

So, what are you going to get in this book? First, I shall take you on a walk down the history lane of hypertension starting from the seventeenth century, giving you a flavour of how we gradually understood this disease, from its humble beginnings to the present day with reference to the digital blood pressure monitor you now have in your home today. It's quite an interesting tour.

Then I move on to give you a foundational understanding of what could be causing your high blood pressure along with a potpourri of surprising things you never knew may be the reason you have the disease and that includes some of the things your doctor may be doing to you in good faith. The benefits of caffeine have been hotly debated in media circles online and offline in the last two decades which is nice and, of course, the effect on blood pressure hasn't evaded this conversation. You will know once and for all whether caffeine is a substance that is worth your while or not if you have high blood pressure with a whole chapter devoted to it.

You may want to know what normal blood pressure is. That will be our next stop, but you will like my descriptive approach on what those blood pressure readings mean in relation to the amount of manual work your heart is doing with different readings. White coat hypertension and masked hypertension do not escape my view. You will have a thorough understanding of both concepts too in more ways than one.

I then provide a reality check on what lifestyle can do for your blood pressure depending on where you are on the complication scale without mincing words. Don't worry, your expectations are respectfully well managed and you will never walk alone no matter how bad it is. If you read a book about high blood pressure and there is no discussion about your kidneys and what role they play, then ask for a refund. The kidneys are central to blood pressure regulation and that dovetails into its management too. You get a whole chapter on that. It's complicated but I simplify it.

Then I get into the meat and potatoes of all the different lifestyle measures available to you. From what you should be eating to exercise, the herbs and spices you need in your life, and a whole chapter devoted to salt. Yes, salt. That controversial essential ingredient in our lives is thoroughly dissected. There is another widely consumed substance that doesn't go unnoticed in this book – alcohol. The relationship between alcohol and high blood pressure is dissected too. How about sleep? I'm sure you would like some exploration on the relationship between sleep and blood pressure control and what to do to get the right amount and quality, wouldn't you? Your needs are taken care of. And, of course, I understand how the word "exercise" sends jitters down your spine. Fear not as I make it simple for you to ease your way into a clever routine that should suit you.

Just before I wrap up this lovely ride, I let you into a little secret of when not to check your blood pressure because you shouldn't on those occasions, and I mean it. The wrap chapter is where I provide you with a mini road map of where to start and what to start with. You will never read a book of mine and be left wondering what you should do next. Not here. You are covered on every level.

Enjoy the ride.

"Healing, just like learning, is a continuous dynamic lifelong journey. Healing is neither a one-time event nor does it follow a linear trajectory. And like any other journey, there will be bumps on the road. It is our duty to scale over those bumps when they appear rather than allow them to halt our progress. The payoff is winning back our health so long as we are stubborn in our pursuit of healing."

Joe Amagada

CHAPTER 1

How Did We Get Here?

In this chapter, I want us to get into the history of hypertension first. Why? Because some of the arguments against managing hypertension were rife historically. Those same arguments are somewhat still in play today. Yes, there are people who believed back then that high blood pressure was a cardiovascular adaptation and best left alone. These were eminent people in the medical field, by the way. You may argue knowledge about hypertension was not profound in that era. However, less than a hundred years ago, eminent figures in the field of medicine like Professor John Hay of University of Liverpool, United Kingdom wrote in 1931:

> "There is some truth in the saying that the greatest danger to a man with a high blood pressure lies in its discovery, because then some fool is certain to try and reduce it."

Professor John was against reduction of blood pressure by "drugs and drastic measures". Although in fairness to him, he also argued quite appropriately for individualisation of care instead of a generic approach. He wasn't opposed to lifestyle modification reading his paper which is a fascinating read, I must say[4a]. He was against the use of drugs, but, at the same time, acknowledged lifestyle modifications could play a role in reducing high blood pressure. Professor John Hay was not alone in this "leave hypertension alone" message. Paul Dudley White, a US Cardiologist had similar views. Views he espoused in 1937 saying:

> "Hypertension may be an important compensatory mechanism which should not be tampered with, even if we were certain that we could control it."[4b]

This belief was so strong, even in this not-so-far-back twentieth century, that a prominent figure like Franklin Roosevelt, who was the president of the United States of America at the time, had his personal physician Admiral Ross McIntire watch the president's blood pressure and health deteriorate over time with a "wait and see" attitude. It is even speculated that President Roosevelt's health was partly responsible for why he allowed Stalin to co-opt a huge part of Eastern Europe into the Soviet Union. That's debatable. What is not debatable though is that at the time of those Yalta negotiations, President Roosevelt's blood pressure was recorded as 260/150 mmHg[4b]. It is commendable Roosevelt was able to even perform basic, personal, or official functions with such blood pressure readings.

That's how pervasive the view was at the time that blood pressure was best left alone as it was deemed a cardiovascular compensatory mechanism. That was then. However, that argument still hangs around today albeit not coming from loud voices. The good news is those preaching that gospel today aren't medical doctors. They are allied medical practitioners. All I will say is the quieter their voices are, the better it is for us. Hypertension is a disease that has the potential to cause extensive damage to target organs when left untouched – and why would you want to? Unless, of course, you subscribe to the opposing view, but you'd be doing that at your own peril. The progressive deterioration of President Roosevelt's health is a classic case of the natural history of hypertension if left unmanaged.

More importantly, it is nice to know how far we have come in the diagnosis and management of hypertension. History will give us a clue. Call it humble beginnings. So, before we dive into the meat and potatoes of this book, it is probably a good idea to delve into a much earlier history of hypertension before the Roosevelt era. After all, if you do not know where you are coming from, you won't know where you are heading. I love history in any context. In fact, I love history so much that if I didn't study medicine, I most probably would have become a historian. I always find history fascinating.

Some of my favourite TV programmes are documentaries based on history. If I am scrolling through the TV channels and I see a history documentary being shown, my scrolling will come to a screeching halt. *Got to watch it*. Past wars. Past leaders. Past interesting personalities. Think King Tutankhamun of Egypt. Past significant events. Think Pompeii and the eruption of Mount Vesuvius. Yes, going that far back to 79 AD fascinates me. The journey of civilisation and industrialisation. You name it. I am in. There is some joy in taking a walk down memory lane. It is good for the soul.

Let me beguile you with a short story to drive home my "history is good for the soul" assertion. There are two ladies. Let us call them Lady A and Lady B. Both are friends. Lady A is super-fit. Lady B, not so much. But Lady B wants to improve her fitness levels too. Credit to her for seeking to do that; she must be encouraged to do so. Lady A arranges for both ladies to go to the gym. On their third visit to the gym, both ladies take the public bus to the gym. Lady B had not eaten prior to the gym visit. Both ladies have a tiring workout. Lady B feels her fit friend pushed her to the point of exhaustion, but she doesn't voice this out to her friend. Anything to please a friend, right?

After the workout session, Lady A insists they walk through a large park to the train station to catch the train home. That would be another two-mile walk to the train station. Two-mile walk to take the train home? Really? This will turn out to be another round of exercise. Call it a top-up session if you like. Not quite what Lady B had in mind.

Annoyingly for Lady B, the bus station, for what should be an easy ride back home, is just a stone's throw away from the gym. A point to highlight is that both ladies took the bus to the gym earlier in the day only because the bus stop was near the gym. Now Lady A wants them to forego that convenience and walk two miles to the train station instead. To please her friend, Lady B agrees even though in her head she is wondering if her weak legs will make it to the train station. Just to add to the mix, Lady B is hungry too. Exhaustion and hunger – not a good combination for an aftermath of what should be a fun activity. Exercise, that is. On their little foot journey through the park, Lady A suggests they sit on the next available park bench for a little chit-chat much to Lady B's pleasure. They do. It is a welcome break for her tired legs. Lady A is whining about her in-laws as they sit watching the world go by.

Whilst Lady A is baring her soul, all Lady B can think of is food. "I need a sandwich and a sugary drink" is the only image swirling around her exhausted mind. Lady B is thinking about food whilst half-listening to her friend when an unkempt gentleman approaches both ladies. This uninvited unkempt gentleman, who interrupted their conversation, is surprisingly well spoken and well mannered. Talk about not judging a book by its cover. Long story short, it turns out this unkempt man has been rendered homeless on account of alcohol abuse. He lost everything. His career. His home. His family. His friends too. But during the conversation both ladies have with this mild-mannered gentleman, he tells them he likes taking a walk through this park ever so often. Because when the going was good, he and his family made frequent visits to the park and every episode of a walk through the park is a "walk down memory lane" for him. It comforts him. It consoles him. It soothes him. Even though he is still struggling with his addiction issues, he finds the walk through the park to be the next best thing to getting him closer to his estranged family. That's the beauty of taking a walk down memory lane. In this case, a walk through the park brings joy and comfort to our alcohol-addicted friend here.

A little journey down memory lane is not only soothing on the soul, but it can also be insightful too. Indeed, for all of us, fond memories can be soul-invigorating. In contrast, we also know one or two historical events that are best confined to the mental archives of history. So, with that little story in mind, let us take a short walk down hypertension memory lane…

Before that though I want to talk about some inventions and how they came about first of all. This will have some relevance to our knowledge and skill regarding measuring blood pressure accurately today shortly. In doing so, you'll get a little insight into how some of the popular discoveries that we know about today – those unrelated to medicine – came about.

My apologies for taking you on a detour. I like inventors and inventions. Inventions tell me someone has been doing a lot of thinking. The inventor has thought of a problem and decided that a solution was possible. Most of us are potential inventors. The difference between us and the real inventors who get patents is that an inventor sees the idea through from original concept to idea actualisation. For the rest of us? Well, we simply dream. We don't do any follow through with our ideas. What a lot of us do not know, though, is a lot of inventions that are granted patents are simply products of refinement. The idea does not have to be clearly original. In most cases, it isn't. Some groundwork would have been done already by someone else and the inventor simply refines the idea or puts finishing touches to the existing concept. And that creates problems for patent lawyers and the courts. A lot of popular inventors got their inventions off the back of some baseline work done previously by one or more individuals.

A classic example of this would be the automated digital blood pressure measuring machines we have today in our homes. These portable automated blood pressure monitoring machines are an off-shoot of the original mercuric sphygmomanometer blood pressure measuring machine that Scipione Riva-Rocci invented from practically nothing in 1896. I shall talk about that some more later in this chapter.

The original inventor stories are quite thin on the ground. Very few of such stories exist. In fact, Mark Lemley of the Stanford Law School says[5]:

"The canonical story of the lone genius inventor is largely a myth. Edison didn't invent the light bulb; he found a bamboo fiber that worked better as a filament in the light bulb developed by Sawyer and Man, who in turn built on lighting work done by others. Bell filed for his telephone patent on the very same day as an independent inventor, Elisha Gray; the case ultimately went to the U.S. Supreme Court, which filled an entire volume of U.S. Reports resolving the question of whether Bell could have a patent despite the fact that he hadn't actually gotten the invention to work at the time he filed.

The Wright Brothers were the first to fly at Kitty Hawk, but their plane didn't work very well, and was quickly surpassed by aircraft built by Glenn Curtis and others – planes that the Wrights delayed by over a decade with patent lawsuits."

Let me shine some more light on this concept of inventors and inventor wars. We know Alexander Graham Bell to be the inventor of the telephone but was he really? Prior to his invention, Philip Reis had built a sound transmitter in 1860. Hermann von Helmholtz was already in the game too having built a receiver[6]. So, here we have a situation where a sound transmitter was already in existence. A receiver already built too. The receiver was just waiting to receive signals. Is there anyone around who could connect these two inventions to the benefit of mankind?

Enter Alexander Graham Bell. What Mr Bell did was to "vary the strength of the current to capture variations in voice and sound", according to Mark Lemley. Graham Bell in his infinite wisdom linked the sound transmitter to the receiver with a fluctuating current that responded to voice and sound. Voilà, an invention was born. Even then, Graham Bell had competition. Elisha Gray had done something similar and filed a patent application on the same day but lost to Graham Bell in the patent court.

Here's another. Before Doctor West's Miracle Toothbrush was invented in 1938, there were toothbrushes around as far back as 1498. Would you believe it? In 1498? Yes, there were. Human beings being the creative beings that we are needed to find a way to deal with smelly breath. These earlier toothbrushes invented in China were made from hog's hairs attached to bones and bamboo[7]. The bones and bamboo were the handles of the toothbrush. They were called boar bristles.

Those boar bristle toothbrushes worked. And why wouldn't they? Anything fluffy that's gentle enough on the gum edges but strong enough to clean the harder teeth is all you need to have a functioning toothbrush if you think about it. Even in primitive societies as of today, the modern toothbrush is not in sight at all. These primitive people simply chew on sticks. You chew on one end of the stick to render it frayed. The frayed end is subsequently employed as the brush for the user's teeth. They clean insanely good. You will be surprised to find out that these chewing sticks are still available on Amazon as we speak. They can't be that bad after all. Dupont de Nemours changed the boar bristles to the modern toothbrush with nylon bristles as we know it today. Now, let's come home to medicine.

If you subscribe to the anti-vaccine ideology, it will annoy you to no end that the first vaccine was invented way back in 1796. Yes, that far back. And I suspect there were no objections to this wonderful invention by Edward Jenner at the time. I could be wrong!

Jenner created molecular material from cowpox, administered it and voilà, generated an immune response to the smallpox virus. Obviously, the process has been refined more and more since then. But an almighty thanks to Edward Jenner for his invention. Some of us would probably not be here today were it not for the outstanding success of the smallpox eradication programme.

Now, let get even closer to home with hypertension. The grandfather to high blood pressure as we know it today in medicine is traceable to a guy by the name of William Harvey. Born in Folkestone, Kent, England on 1st April 1578, William was an outstanding physician of the seventeenth century. To be a personal physician to two different Kings of England is no small feat. This feat may indicate an element of smartness or just being a lucky guy. I'd like to think the former rather than the latter. William Harvey was a personal physician to King James I from February 1618 and later, in 1632, became personal physician to King Charles I. In fact, he went on voyages with King Charles at the time[8].

William Harvey was one of those who pushed back against widely held beliefs about witchcraft in those archaic times. It's nice to see well-read individuals speak against beliefs that were not just popular but dangerous at the same time even if no one else did. These were beliefs that put lives and freedom at risk. William did not just challenge the witchcraft tenet but went as far as producing evidence that would secure the release of individuals accused of witchcraft. But it's not his work in the unhinged world of witchcraft that interests us here. Rather it is his work in the field of anatomy and physiology that impresses me the most. William is practically one of the first people to lay the groundwork for blood circulation as we know it today.

Prior to William Harvey's ground-breaking work, Claudius Galenus (anglicised as Galen) had proposed that the arterial and venous systems were separate. But incorrectly that the two systems (venous and arterial) connected through openings (or pores) between the right ventricle and the left ventricle. The right and left ventricles are the bigger chambers of the heart. These connecting openings, as proposed by Galen, were not visible to the naked eye. You could liken Galen's theory of circulation to the sweat pores in our skin. You can't see them, but you know they are there. The evidence being that you sweat when you are hot. In the case of the pores between the ventricles of the heart, the evidence being the difference in the colour of blood from the right side and the left side. It is hard to imagine that theory was believed at the time knowing what we know now about oxygenated blood and deoxygenated blood. Anyway, that view held sway for a long time until William Harvey came along.

The venous system at the time was called the "natural system" and the arterial side was labelled the "vital system". The natural system arose from the liver and the vital system was deemed very essential because it breathed life and heat into all body tissues. The vital system contained the blood of life and spirits.

What was also theorised at the time was that there had to be a cooling system if the arterial blood contained heat and distributed the heat therein. The cooling system identified were the lungs. You could say the lungs provided the elixir of life because if there was nothing to cool the blood down, then the body would overheat. Maybe we die of heat exhaustion in the absence of the lungs when you think about the prevailing theory at the time. Thank heavens for the lungs. The logic is not hard to see. If something sucked in air from the outside, then the air must perform some function in the lungs – cooling. The existing theory projected lungs as the fan or air conditioning system. These were popularly held views in the scientific world at the time. And these views prevailed for centuries. So, if you wanted to stick a knife into these beliefs, you had better be good. And have your facts as solid as a rock.

William Harvey had these. He was prepared for the fight. Mainly because he had been experimenting on animals. Cold-blooded animals were his experimental tools if you like. He had conviction in the results of his experiments. Even when you are convinced about your discovery and you are about to shatter pre-held strong beliefs, you will still approach your publication with trepidation. Wolves in the world of medicine and science didn't emerge in the twentieth and twenty-first centuries. They have always been around, and they will eat you and your reputation up in a slow and steady manner. So much so that William Harvey was to share his anticipated fear like this:

"But what remains to be said about the quantity and source of the blood which thus passes, is of so novel and unheard-of character that I not only fear injury to myself from the envy of a few, but I tremble lest I have mankind at large for my enemies, so much doth want and custom, that become as another nature, and doctrine once sown and that hath struck deep root, and respect for antiquity, influence all men : still the die is cast, and my trust is in my love of truth, and the candour that inheres in cultivated minds."

William Harvey found his experimentation complex and almost gave up on it to just go along with the existing dictum as proposed by Galen and others. But he had a call of duty. He persisted. He felt the existing theory was wrong and needed to push ahead with his scientific work. His persistence paid off. William Harvey was the first to really connect the dots about how blood circulated in the body. William noticed that when the heart contracted, the left bigger chamber of the heart – the left ventricle – generated a pulse in our arteries. He felt a pulsation peripherally when the heart contracted. William also established that the bigger chamber on the right side of the heart – the right ventricle – delivered blood to the lungs. William noticed that the right and left ventricles moved together at the same time. Prior to his discovery, it was thought the right ventricle and left ventricle contracted separately. The preceding theory was that the two ventricles were independent of each other.

William didn't stop there. What we now know as heart rate, which is how many times your heart beats per minute, was one of William Harvey's discoveries too. He also did a calculation of how much blood the heart pumps out with each beat. In medicine, we call that stroke volume. By extension, he attempted the calculation of the ejection fraction. This is basically the percentage of blood the ventricles push out from their current volume at rest. When your heart is failing, which is one of the complications of long-standing hypertension, the ejection fraction gets lower and lower as your condition worsens because the heart muscle is tired from doing too much "heavy lifting" pumping out blood against a high resistance when your blood pressure is high. All of these are the product of William Harvey's discoveries published in his 72-page book titled *Exercitatio Anatomica de Motu Cordis et Sanguinis in Animalibus*. As anticipated, William Harvey's work was met with stiff opposition and even ridicule. Yes, scientists were nasty even then. It didn't start today. Expect opposition and a thorough dissection of your work if you are planning to make a paradigm shift. You are essentially telling your predecessors that they have been wrong all along. Why would you expect an easy ride? That's not going to happen.

In the world of inventions and discoveries, when you make a breakthrough, you should expect some sort of defence either in the law courts for patents (if there are competing interests) as we saw earlier or in the courts of scientific opinion. The court of scientific opinion can be just as brutal. As it happens, William Harvey was right, and we owe a lot about what we now know as the cardiovascular system today to his diligence and persistence in understanding how the heart works, how the arteries work and how the venous system works. So, now that we are clear about how the circulatory system works, thanks to Harvey, could we measure the pressure in the circulatory system? More specifically, the arterial tree.

Enter Stephen Hales[9]. Born in Bekesbourne, Kent, England on 17th September 1677, Stephen Hales was another eminent and luminous scientist. He was luminous because his work covered a lot of ground and this includes the fields of chemistry, physiology and even botany. Stephen Hales hailed (no pun intended) from a large family but that did not stop him from attending a prestigious college, the Corpus Christi College, Cambridge. Yes, Cambridge University has been around for that long just in case you were wondering. William Harvey also got his medical doctorate degree from Cambridge University.

Stephen Hales obtained degrees in philosophy, classics, mathematics, and natural sciences. That's quite a collection of degrees. Heaven knows if he had any social life at all in his university days. The year 1703 was a particularly good year for Stephen Hales because in that year, he obtained his master's degree and was also ordained as a deacon in Cambridgeshire. Stephen Hales was someone who had a very inquisitive mind. He was obsessed with experimentation. In fact, he drew condemnation from a lot of his colleagues including his friends because he experimented a lot on animals. Hear Alexander Pope, a friend of his:

> "He commits most of these barbarities with the thought of its being of use to man. But how do we know that we have a right to kill creatures that we are so little above as dogs, for our curiosity, or even for some use to us?"

So, as you can see from the above, the debate about animal rights has been going on for hundreds of years. It's nothing new. Stephen Hales labelled his works *Statical Essays*. In his *Haemastaticks,* he described the experiments he had been conducting on animals. Stephen Hales was obsessed with animal physiology. Of interest to us was his work on how to measure the "force of blood". This is what we now know as blood pressure. During his experimentation, Stephen Hales would insert tubes into arteries of animals and observe how high the column of blood rose when the heart ventricles contracted[10]. This was how we got our first understanding of the force of blood in arteries. This is what today represents blood pressure and Stephen Hales was the first person to describe this phenomenon in 1733. Stephen Hales did not stop there. He also did some ghastly experimentation on animals by bleeding them to death and, at the same time, observing the blood pressure changes as the animals bled gradually. Obviously, this was very distressing to his close friends and colleagues. Hence Alexander Pope was forced to make that comment about his friend.

As cruel as it appears to all animal lovers, Hales was the first person that enabled our understanding of the physiological changes that occur when there is a progressive loss of blood. This is basically exsanguination. What Hales observed in animals is exactly the same thing that happens in humans when we experience heavy blood loss either quickly or gradually. As part of his work, Hales unsuccessfully came up with a technique to dissolve bladder stones. It didn't work. His failure at bladder stone dissolution led him to a further discovery. He designed forceps for the removal of bladder stones instead and at the same time also designed a bladder catheter to drain urine out of the bladder[11].

It may also interest you that Stephen Hales, through his experimentation, correctly described the functions of the valves of the left side of the heart: the mitral valves and the aortic valves. Stephen Hales was the first scientist to postulate that blood pressure was the result of friction of blood flow in the smaller arteries in our body. This is what we now call peripheral resistance. Indeed, peripheral resistance is blood pressure really. The higher the resistance downstream, the higher your blood pressure and vice versa. That's how industrious Stephen Hales was. And a big thumbs up to Stephen for his work and more importantly correct interpretations.

There wasn't a lot of movement in the field of hypertension after William Harvey's and Stephen Hales' discoveries until the year 1808 when Thomas Young gave a description of the pathology of hypertension. In 1836, Richard Bright noted that some of his patients who had kidney disease also had an enlarged heart but the link with hypertension was not identified at the time. Despite the work done by Stephen Hale in the eighteenth century, we still had no device to measure blood pressure in humans until 1896 when Scipione Riva-Rocci discovered the sphymomanometer[12]. Finally, we had an instrument with which we could measure blood pressure clinically.

But having the sphygmomanometer was not enough. Measuring blood pressure reliably was of the utmost importance. Enter Nikolai Korotkoff[13]. Remember when I said discoveries don't have to be original from the ground up. Graham Bell and the telephone "invention" comes to mind. Sometimes what a smart inventor does is simply take on someone else's baseline idea and build on it. That's what Nikolai Koroktoff did. He polished up and advanced Scipione Riva-Rocci's earlier discovery. Sometimes in medicine, and science in general, making your point doesn't have to command verbosity. You can make your point succinctly. In his presentation to the Imperial Military Academy, Koroktoff said the following:

"The cuff of Riva-Rocci is placed on the middle third of the upper arm; the pressure within the cuff is quickly raised up to complete cessation of circulation below the cuff. Then, letting the mercury of the manometer fall one listens to the artery just below the cuff with a children's stethoscope. At first no sounds are heard. With the falling of the mercury in the manometer down to a certain height, the first short tones appear; their appearance indicates the passage of part of the pulse wave under the cuff. It follows that the manometric figure at which the first tone appears corresponds to the maximal pressure. With the further fall of the mercury in the manometer one hears the systolic compression murmurs, which pass again into tones (second). Finally, all sounds disappear. The time of the cessation of sounds indicates the free passage of the pulse wave; in other words at the moment of the disappearance of the sounds the minimal blood pressure within the artery predominates over the pressure in the cuff. It follows that the manometric figures at this time correspond to the minimal blood pressure."

Did you like that? I hope you did because that description remains the cornerstone of blood pressure measurement today. The aneroid blood pressure machines which later became popular because of the bulkiness of the Koroktoff mercuric sphygmomanometer use the same technology. Even now, the shiny digital blood pressure monitors that we all have at home rely on the same principle. The only difference is the digital machines use oscillometric technology to detect the flow of blood through the artery in which the blood pressure is being measured. Some things never change!

By the way, it wasn't until 1981 that the fully automated oscillometric sphygmomanometer was invented by Donald Nunn. Another off-shoot invention of the Scipione Riva-Rocci prototype of 1896. That Koroktoff presentation was made in the year 1905. What Koroktoff described in that meeting to the uninitiated, (and I am referring to non-medics reading this book) is that the first sound represents the systolic blood pressure (upper value) and the point where the sounds disappear on the stethoscope represent the diastolic blood pressures (bottom value). You don't need to know that fine details anyway. That's for us doctors and nurses to chew on.

What is noteworthy here is that from a haphazard approach in the preceding centuries, we now have a standard instrument and a standard way of measuring blood pressure. This is all thanks to Koroktoff. This is how science evolves. And this is what I love about discoveries and inventions. Now you know why I told you earlier on in the chapter that I love inventors. Hopefully, you, reading this book, will become one of them. I'm counting on you to come up with something revolutionary even if it is a spin-off of someone else's idea.

So, what has happened since the Koroktoff discovery? Have we moved the needle further to enhance the management of high blood pressure? Maybe. But have the patients with high blood pressure been impressed with treatment methods? That's debatable. From the time of Koroktoff, we have tried various treatment options. We sailed from the performance of sympathectomy in the 1920s into the sea of the rice diet in the 1940s. Sympathectomy is a procedure which aims at interrupting and eliminating the flow of nerve impulse in the sympathetic nervous system. This can be achieved either surgically or chemically.

Chemical agents like guanethidine and bretylium designed to reduce sympathetic nerve impulse flow were introduced in place of surgical sympathectomy[14], because surgical sympathectomy demonstrated unacceptable untoward collateral damage. Chemical sympathectomy wasn't any better either. Even anti-malarials, like pentaquine, have been tried. The success rates of a lot of the treatment methods, especially the earlier ones, have been less than impressive.

The development and introduction of medications that enable you to pee a lot more in the late 1950s was a significant landmark in the management of high blood pressure. An example of these medications is hydrochlorothiazide. These medications belong to a group called diuretics. Along with this was also the introduction of hydralazine medication. The fact we still use these medications in the management of high blood pressure currently is a testament to their relative effectiveness and tolerability. A lot of medications and treatment modalities have come and faded away as quickly as they were introduced. This is largely because of either ineffectiveness or having side effects that made the hypertensive patient worse in other aspects of their overall health.

Hypertension is a disease that has been extensively studied. But despite all the resources that have gone into hypertension research, we are still at a loss as to the cause of this disease in a vast majority of the sufferers, although we have a bunch of risk factors to guide us. Sometimes the cause is readily found on investigation but in most patients no obvious cause is identified, and these cases fall into the classification called essential hypertension.

Now, we have a huge portfolio of medications to manage high blood pressure which in a way is a good thing. But as most people with high blood pressure will attest, success rates even with newer medications is still incredibly low. But we have come a long way from the seventeenth century when the understanding of circulation by William Harvey was made available to us to the present time where we are still floundering in terms of effective treatments without intolerable side effects.

The ideal treatment would be one that lowers blood pressure and has, at the same time, few and tolerable side effects. The main reason why people seek alternative therapy is the issue of side effects of blood pressure medications. Hypertensive individuals do not want to be left with side effects that make their lives miserable. They are therefore justified in seeking alternative solutions that give them results with little or no side effects. Fair deal, I think. So long as that transition is not executed in a reckless manner.

You need not worry though. You will be ahead of the game in managing your high blood pressure with lifestyle measures by the time you have completed reading this book. That is a promise from me to you.

CHAPTER 2

What Causes High Blood Pressure?

No one likes the diagnosis of hypertension or any other disease for that matter. We would rather be well and happy and be completely free of disease. But in life we can't always get what we want. This means some of us end up carrying a disease burden. Hypertension is one of such diseases. Naturally, when someone gets a diagnosis of hypertension, one of the first questions they ask their doctor is: what caused my high blood pressure? The problem is the answer is not always obvious, at least not in the beginning anyway. So, for the most part, your doctor will not be able to provide a concrete answer to your question at your first meeting. What this means is, when a diagnosis of hypertension is made, that triggers a chain of events. One of which is a process of investigation to find out why you have hypertension. Sometimes clinical and laboratory investigations will not provide the answer to the question as to why you have developed high blood pressure. But it behoves on your doctor to carry out those investigations in the hope of finding the cause regardless.

That's usually a starting point. The reason behind investigating is, when a cause is found, the management of the hypertension can also be directed at that cause. If a cause is not found, we generally will say you have "essential hypertension". I'm not sure how the label of "essential" came about because it sort of suggests that the disease, hypertension, is somehow essential in someone's life. I don't think so. Hypertension is not essential in anyone's life. That is not a particularly good name, in my humble opinion. I prefer the term primary hypertension, but it is rarely used by doctors. We seem to prefer the former.

In searching for a possible cause of high blood pressure, it is important to bear in mind that only 5–10% of hypertensive individuals will have an identifiable cause[15]. In these individuals, we usually say they have secondary hypertension. Whilst it may be an advantage to have secondary hypertension, the treatment, however, is not always easy. So, individuals with secondary hypertension may have something to point the finger at but that does not always translate into easy management. These individuals still face some of the management difficulties that those with essential hypertension also experience.

But it is a lot easier to have a focal point or a lever to pull on when dealing with a problem as opposed to flailing aimlessly in the dark, as is the case with essential hypertension. So, from that perspective it is probably arguably better to have secondary hypertension as you can direct treatment at the cause. Whether one is successful or not at treating secondary hypertension is another matter altogether but at least you have a target to aim at. A bullseye if you like. Now, let's look at some of the possible causes of secondary hypertension.

The Kidneys

Long standing kidney disease of any kind can potentially result in hypertension. The kidneys and high blood pressure have a circuitous relationship. Any disease of the kidney that affects the filtration system will lead to high blood pressure.

Additionally, if the kidneys are damaged by repeated kidney infections over a good number of years, that would lead to some kidney damage and loss of functionality which may result in hypertension in the later years.

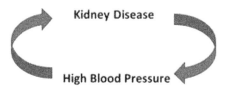

Figure 1

As you can see from Figure 1 above, kidney disease tends to lead to high blood pressure and high blood pressure causes kidney disease too. This relationship between kidney disease and hypertension is not always straightforward. We aren't always sure which one came first. Did the kidney disease cause the hypertension or did the high blood pressure cause the kidney disease? So, we end up with the chicken and the egg situation.

Speaking in broad terms, however, longstanding kidney diseases will usually result in high blood pressure. For instance, a condition we call glomerulonephritis in which the filters in the kidneys become inflamed and subsequently become damaged will lead to high blood pressure. And this includes other diseases that target the kidneys as part of their complication network. I am looking at you, lupus and diabetes. Yes, these two diseases cause hypertension through their kidney damage too.

The Adrenal Glands

The adrenal glands are two tiny organs that sit on top of the kidneys on both sides. There are certain diseases of the adrenal glands that result in high blood pressure. One such disease is

Cushing syndrome where you have excessive production of the hormone, cortisol. High levels of cortisol circulating in your body will lead to high blood pressure. About 85% of cases of Cushing syndrome have their origin in the brain or more specifically in the pituitary gland[16]. Patients with Cushing syndrome will have other symptoms, such as a moon-like face, glucose intolerance, dry skin, lots of belly fat and brittle bones amongst other features.

Another adrenal condition that causes high blood pressure is what we refer to as pheochromocytoma. Yes, it is a tongue-twister, I know. Pheochromocytoma is usually the result of a tumour arising from the inner aspects (the core) of the adrenal glands[17]. These tumours are usually benign meaning they are non-cancerous. In this condition, the adrenal glands produce excessive amounts of catecholamines. Catecholamines are hormones, more specifically adrenaline and noradrenaline which you are most likely familiar with. High levels of adrenaline and noradrenaline will certainly push up your blood pressure levels which by definition is hypertension. Apart from raising your blood pressure, individuals with pheochromocytoma will also experience a fast heartbeat, along with episodes of sudden onset anxiety symptoms like nervousness, sweating and headaches. The usual panic attack symptoms.

Another condition of the adrenal gland that causes hypertension is hyperaldosteronism. This is a condition in which the adrenal glands produce excess aldosterone hormone. This condition is usually caused by a small tumour on the outer aspects of the adrenal gland[18]. High levels of aldosterone in the body will result in excessive retention of salt and water which increases the blood volume and results in hypertension. The problem here is that whilst the aldosterone conserves sodium in the body through the kidneys, it also results in the loss of potassium from the body through urine. This is not good as you need your potassium to lower your blood pressure.

The Thyroid Gland

The thyroid gland produces the hormone thyroxine. Thyroxine influences the function of the heart and the circulatory system. What this means is excessive production of thyroxine, or too little production of thyroxine, will influence your blood pressure. So, both hypothyroidism, which is an under-active thyroid (meaning too little thyroxine present in the body) and hyperthyroidism, which is an over-active thyroid (where we have excessive production of thyroxine) can cause hypertension.

There is also a secondary effect of the hormone thyroxine. It influences cholesterol levels too. This is an indirect effect through the process of cholesterol metabolism. Anything that influences cholesterol deposition on our blood vessel wall will, over time, cause a hardening of the vessel wall with the result of a rise in blood pressure.

The Pancreas

The pancreas makes the hormone insulin and glucagon amongst others. What concerns us here is the hormone insulin. When the pancreas makes too little insulin or none at all, the end result is diabetes. Diabetes is a disorder of glucose metabolism. Any situation where there is an abnormal glucose metabolism involving high sugar levels in the blood circulation is a recipe for abnormal cholesterol metabolism too. Have you ever wondered why people with insulin resistance (i.e. type 2 diabetes) struggle with their blood lipids? That's the reason. Persistently high circulating sugar levels lead to abnormal lipids in the blood because the liver has no choice but to convert some of the sugar presented to it into lipids like triglycerides, LDL cholesterol and other fatty acids. These two conditions are part of the metabolic syndrome, as they seem to occur simultaneously if left untreated.

Speaking of insulin resistance, the mechanism of the disease process is somewhat different. Here is what happens. The pancreas may do its job by producing enough insulin in response to the sugar in circulation, but if the target cells – which are the muscle cells – and the liver cells are unresponsive to the action of insulin then we will have high blood sugar levels. The reason for this is that the target cells are supposed to open their doors to let the sugar in from the blood circulation. That's how blood sugar gets lowered. However, in insulin resistance, the target cells shut their doors to circulating blood glucose. This failure to let the sugar have access to the target cells results in the sugar being abandoned in the blood circulation and blood sugar levels remain high.

Here's how the process is supposed to work. You have a meal. The carbohydrates in the meal get broken down to simple sugars like glucose. The glucose gets absorbed and blood glucose rises as a result. The pancreas responds to a rise in blood glucose by releasing insulin. Insulin knocks on the door of the target cell. The target cell responds to the signals from the insulin and opens its door. Glucose glides inside the cell from the blood circulation. As more of the target cells obey commands from the insulin, more glucose exits the blood circulation into the liver cells and muscle cells (the main target cells).

More glucose exiting the circulation into these target cells results in lower blood glucose. If this mechanism fails, i.e. the target cells don't obey the call from insulin to open their doors, the glucose from your meals remains floating in the blood and blood glucose levels remain high as a result. This is what we call insulin resistance: the cells are resisting the call from insulin to open their doors.

With glucose levels remaining high from this resistance, the pancreas responds by releasing more insulin into the circulation hoping for better obedience by the target cells next time around. Alas, that doesn't happen. Instead, you end up with high blood sugar levels *and* high blood insulin levels too. Classic insulin resistance!

Your insulin levels will remain high even when you haven't had your first meal of the day in the morning because your blood sugar is equally high. This is the fasted state. Ideally, your insulin and blood sugar levels should be at their lowest before your first meal of the day. High fasting insulin levels and high fasting blood sugar levels are classical insulin resistance.

There is a particularly strong association between insulin resistance and hypertension. As stated earlier, the hallmarks of insulin resistance are elevated fasting insulin levels and high fasting blood sugar. These two parameters are markers to look out for when attempting to make a diagnosis of insulin resistance.

If you go digging for the existence of insulin resistance in a lot of patients with high blood pressure, you will find it. You just need to look. One study[19] looked at fifty individuals with hypertension and matched them for age and sex with another fifty individuals without hypertension. For the study, the researchers measured blood levels of fasting insulin as well as their fasting blood sugar levels. What they found was that there was a statistically significant difference in the mean fasting blood glucose levels between the two groups. The fasting blood glucose levels were higher in the group with hypertension compared to the group without hypertension. A similar result was also found with fasting blood insulin levels; there were significantly higher fasting insulin levels in the group with hypertension.

A meta-analysis pools different studies from different authors together so long as the authors have similar or near similar study objectives on the same topic. One such meta-analysis[20] that looked at over 55,000 individuals from eleven studies showed that high fasting insulin levels – which we see in insulin resistance patients – increase your risk of developing high blood pressure by 54%. The study authors concluded that:

"Elevated fasting insulin concentrations or insulin resistance as estimated by homeostasis model assessment is independently associated with an exacerbated risk of hypertension in the general population. Early intervention of hyperinsulinemia or insulin resistance may help clinicians to identify the high risk of hypertensive population."

Hyperinsulinemia refers to high insulin levels in the blood. A combination of hypertension and insulin resistance does have a negative impact on the function of the heart. Do we have any scientific proof for that? Of course, we do.

This scientific study[21] looked at 704 individuals from a community with a high prevalence of hypertension and obesity. The researchers assessed cardiac function using echocardiogram. The emphasis was to study the functionality of the left lower chamber – the left ventricle – in the presence of high blood pressure and insulin resistance. They found out that the left ventricle was more likely to function poorly when individuals had a combination of high blood pressure and insulin resistance compared to individuals who had normal blood pressure. We know that the function of the left side of the heart which distributes blood into the arterial tree is negatively affected by hypertension which is the reason we want to control high blood pressure in the first place. What that piece of research tells us is that this problem of a poorly performing left ventricle is made worse when an individual has a combination of hypertension and insulin resistance. Further, it tells us that, by extension, a combination of insulin resistance and hypertension is more likely to lead to heart failure in the long term if both conditions are poorly controlled.

By the way, poorly controlled diabetes, whether it is type 1 or type 2, will always target the kidneys as an organ. When diabetes does that to your kidneys, you wind up with what we call diabetic nephropathy. Diabetic nephropathy is the term we use to describe the destructive effect of diabetes on the structure and function of the kidneys. Diabetic nephropathy is nearly always associated with high blood pressure.

Sleep Apnoea

In sleep apnoea, the muscles around your throat become lax during sleep and this leads to interruption of your breathing temporarily. Obviously when this happens, your breathing is obstructed, and this is what we call obstructive sleep apnoea. Some of the symptoms of obstructive sleep apnoea will include breathing stopping and restarting, making funny noises during sleep like snorting, choking, or gasping, having fragmented sleep and, of course, loud snoring.

You may wake up with a headache or feeling tired and lethargic during the day. You could also have problems with concentration which will affect your problem-solving skills at work. You may feel nervous and irritable which could affect your relationships at work and at home. All of these are not helpful for a normal blood pressure. Poor sleep, regardless of the cause, will lead to high levels of stress hormones in the morning, in particular cortisol. Not only that, there will be a rise of adrenaline and noradrenaline when you sleep poorly. The combination of unusually high levels of cortisol, adrenaline and noradrenaline is the recipe for high blood pressure. Therefore, taking steps to deal with sleep apnoea should be a matter of priority in all individuals with obstructive sleep apnoea. If you don't resolve your sleep apnoea, your blood pressure medications won't get very far controlling your blood pressure.

Autoimmune Diseases

Autoimmune diseases can also be a cause of high blood pressure, mainly because these diseases target multiple organs, including the kidneys. A good example of an autoimmune disease is systemic lupus. Lupus is a systemic autoimmune disease that occurs when our immune system attacks different organs. Such organs could include the joints, the skin, the kidneys, the blood cells and even the heart and lungs.

As you will have learnt earlier in this chapter, any condition like lupus that targets the kidneys is most likely going to lead to kidney damage. Once the kidneys are damaged, the filtration system of the kidneys is affected, which will ultimately result in a loss of functionality with high blood pressure being the ultimate consequence.

What About Essential Hypertension?

As stated earlier, essential hypertension is one where we do not really have a known cause for it. But there are certain factors that will put you at risk of developing essential hypertension. These are what we call risk factors. The rule is the more risk factors you have, the higher the likelihood that you will develop hypertension. But I have always said this: having one or more risk factors does not mean you should resign yourself to that destiny. Having multiple risk factors shouldn't mean you are definitely going to develop high blood pressure. You will if you quietly accept the risk factors and wait for the hypertension to arrive. Because it most certainly will happen if you do nothing about it.

The beauty of outlining your individual risk factors is that you can identify whether or not you are at risk. What then needs to happen is for you to take steps to deal with any modifiable risk factors you might have. Risk factors are usually divided into "modifiable" and "non-modifiable". Non-modifiable risk factors are the ones that we cannot do anything about. They are here to stay. But you can still do your best to mitigate the risks posed by the non-modifiable risk factors. The picture gets better with modifiable risk factors though. These are the risk factors that you *can* influence; sometimes not very easily, but it's doable all the same. To be frank, there is no excuse for you to not take steps to mitigate the dangers from modifiable risk factors. The only thing stopping you is a lack of awareness and a lack of desire to do what is necessary.

But that is why you are reading this book. Because, like they say, knowledge is power. Once you know about the risk factors that are within your power to mitigate then you have every right to exercise those powers. Doing what is within your power means you significantly reduce your risk of developing that health problem. In this instance, we are talking about high blood pressure, a condition that has the potential to cause significant disability and even death.

So, with that said, what are the risk factors for hypertension? Below is the list:

- Smoking
- Being overweight or obese
- Lack of physical activity or being sedentary
- Too much stress at home or at work or both

- Alcohol abuse
- Age (or should I say getting older) – 65 and over
- Family history of high blood pressure
- Consuming too much salt in your diet
- Being of African descent (and, of course, that includes Afro-Caribbeans and African Americans)
- Sleep deprivation
- Not eating enough fruits and vegetables
- Economic deprivation

Looking at the list of risk factors above, getting older, having a family history of high blood pressure and being of African descent are examples of non-modifiable risk factors. As you can see, there isn't a lot you can do about these risk factors. Hence, they are referred to as non-modifiable. But the positive side to this is that being aware of any non-modifiable risk factors you have should provide you with inspiration to take active steps in doing what is necessary for the prevention of hypertension.

The point I am making here is that *awareness* of non-modifiable risk factors should push you in the direction of prevention. This is all about self-care. Most people who have non-modifiable risk factors also have one or two modifiable risk factors unless they are lucky. What you do in either case does not differ. You should take the same steps for non-modifiable risk factors as you would for modifiable risk factors for hypertension. If you want to prevent hypertension – or manage the disease if you already have it – the actions required are essentially the same.

There is no distinction between the steps you take both for prevention and for self-management of hypertension. In this book, I will emphasise all the things you need to do to lower your blood pressure. But let me say this: if you want to prevent high blood pressure, then you must do the things people with high blood pressure are supposed to do. If you take steps to do what helps hypertensives control their blood pressure, then you will prevent it if you do not have it already. The salient takeaway here is that both the prevention and the management are essentially the same. The only difference is implementing the steps for self-management for the purpose of prevention puts you well ahead of the curve. You are essentially taking the bull by the horns which means hypertension will not be knocking on your door anytime soon.

It is the same advice that I give to people who are trying to prevent type 2 diabetes. I simply tell them, if you want to prevent type 2 diabetes, just eat, and adopt the health behaviours of a diabetic. It's that simple. The same applies to the prevention of hypertension. If you want to prevent hypertension, then adopt the behaviours of someone with well-controlled hypertension. Simply make the same behavioural changes in your life.

Prescription

For those with secondary hypertension, all of your efforts should be directed at tackling the identified secondary cause of your hypertension. For instance, if you have sleep apnoea, you must do everything you can to resolve it in order to get better blood pressure readings. Because if you ignore that basic advice, you will be chasing shadows for a good while yet. That's the recipe for success for reversing secondary hypertension.

For individuals with primary hypertension (essential hypertension), look at the risk factors list I have provided above. Pick the risk factors that apply to you and get to work. Focus on resolving the modifiable risk factors and worry less about the non-modifiable ones.

Obsessing and whining over the non-modifiable ones only leads to frustration and stress, both of which will not help your blood pressure readings. Let me reiterate: concentrate your efforts on the modifiable risk factors. More about this later.

CHAPTER 3

Surprising Causes of High Blood Pressure

In this section of the book, we are going to be talking about some of the things we do quite innocently that may be contributing to our hypertension. But this problem is not confined to the things that we do as individuals. Your doctor may also be contributing to the problem.

Some of the medications your doctor may be prescribing for you may inadvertently cause your blood pressure to rise. Indeed, the purpose of this section of the book is to alert you to some of these things that either you or your doctor may be doing that impact your blood pressure and your blood pressure control negatively. It is quite possible that both you and your personal physician may be sabotaging your blood pressure control efforts or just plainly causing hypertension unknowingly.

So, becoming aware of these things that I'm going to be talking about in this section of the book would bring that much needed awareness of these products. Meaning you could either stop using these products altogether or alter the way you use them. The ideal thing to do would be to look for substitutes.

If you search far enough, you will usually find substitutes somehow. It may take thinking outside of the box to come up with alternatives for some of the products you may be using, but they do exist. Some of these products will surprise you, as they appear very innocent and are often popular.

So, let us talk about these products.

Painkillers

Quite a number of the painkillers available both on prescription and over the counter can make your blood pressure control difficult. The main culprits here are the nonsteroidal anti-inflammatory medications and the drugs we call cyclooxygenase-2 (cox-2) enzyme inhibitors. The problem with this group of medications is that they have a not-so-pleasant effect on kidney function when you use them. And as you recall from the earlier issues that we discussed in the preceding chapter, anything that affects the smooth functioning of the kidneys will have either an indirect or direct effect on blood pressure control.

And guess what. If you don't have hypertension already, there's research evidence (which I will reference below) to support the view that chronic use of these medications could predispose the individual to a diagnosis of hypertension over time. So, these groups of medications not only make blood pressure control difficult, they also can cause hypertension when used in the long term.

The way these nonsteroidal anti-inflammatory medications and cox-2 inhibitors raise blood pressure is through salt and water retention in the kidneys and they also appear to have a direct effect on the relaxation of the walls of our arteries making them stiffer. These medications do this by inhibiting the activity of the cyclooxygenase-2 enzyme that helps in the production of prostaglandins that ordinarily will relax blood vessels[22]. The problems associated with these medications are worse in patients who have diabetes alongside hypertension. In fact, in some of these patients, weight gain and swelling of the feet may accompany chronic use of these medications. This is a direct result of fluid retention from salt conservation in the kidneys.

This effect on the kidneys is not confined only to people with hypertension. There is research evidence to suggest that chronic users of nonsteroidal anti-inflammatory medications have a 40% increase in risk of receiving a diagnosis of hypertension compared to non-users[23]. This is serious when we consider that these medications are widely used in the population. Using these nonsteroidal anti-inflammatory agents and cox-2 inhibitor medications alongside ACE inhibitors blood pressure medications (like ramipril or lisinopril), beta blockers (like labetalol, atenolol or bisoprolol), and diuretics (like indapamide or hydrochlorothiazide) gives any cardiovascular complications considerable significance. Why? Because bundling these painkillers with ACE inhibitors, beta blockers or diuretics results in a worsened outcome. This constitutes a public health concern, particularly considering 12 million US citizens take these nonsteroidal anti-inflammatory medications alongside blood pressure medications[24]. The worst offenders amongst this group of medications are:

- Indomethacin (Indocin, Indocin SR, Tivorbex)
- Naproxene (Aleve, Anaprox, Naprelan, Anaprox, Anaprox DS, Aflaxen)
- Piroxicam (Feldene)
- Rofecoxib (Vioxx, Ceoxx, Ceeoxx) – withdrawn from the market

Others include:

- Diclofenac (Cambia, Cataflam, Voltaren XR, Zipsor, Zorvolex)
- Ibuprofen (Motrim, Advil, Neurofen,)
- Ketoprofen (Orudis, Orudis KT, Oruvail)
- Oxaprozin (Daypro)
- Celecoxib (Celebrex)

So, as you can see from above, these rather innocent-looking medications we use often aren't so harmless after all when you consider their cardiovascular implications.

St John's Wort

The fact St John's Wort is a popular product all over the world is not in doubt. In fact, St John's Wort outsells the main conventional antidepressants in the US. The reason behind the popularity of St John's Wort is based on a 1996 meta-analysis study[25] that looked at twenty-three randomised control trials involving 1757 patients with mild to moderately severe depression. The study concluded that St John's Wort was more effective than placebo for the treatment of mild to moderate depressive disorders.

The active ingredient in St John's Wort is hypericin. Not surprisingly, St John's Wort is made up of hypericin extracts. More recent studies, however, have shown conflicting results, but this hasn't stopped the sales of St John's Wort heading north. St John's Wort is one of the most investigated non-pharmacological products available today. So, how does St John's Wort contribute to high blood pressure?

Research evidence suggests that St John's Wort is an inhibitor of the monoamine oxidase enzyme which leads to the accumulation of serotonin, dopamine and noradrenaline[26]. Accumulation of these substances in the brain has the potential to render the user excitable. Excitability has a negative impact on blood pressure.

The potential problem with St John's Wort and its contribution to high blood pressure becomes significant when an individual combines it with tyramine-rich foods like cheese, sauerkraut, chicken liver, red wine, and soy sauce, amongst others. Using these foods alongside St John's Wort can result in hypertensive crisis.

Indeed, there is this case report of a 41-year-old gentleman[27] who was taking St John's Wort. On this eventful day, he felt he needed a relaxation snack. So, he ate cheese and had a glass of red wine to quell his cravings. The highlight of his afternoon snack was a hypertensive crisis that needed management in the emergency department. This should be a warning for anybody who is taking St John's Wort to be careful, as the potential for dangerously high blood pressure is real if you consume the tyramine-rich foods listed previously. It is a mistake that is very easily made.

Liquorice (Licorice)

Want to know if liquorice consumption can lead to hypertension? Let me acquaint you with this case of a 45-year-old lady who was looking for substitutes for caffeinated teas and settled for liquorice tea instead[28]. She had been using the liquorice tea for a couple of weeks when she developed symptoms of sweating, headaches, and hot flashes. She went to see her doctor who checked her blood pressure and noticed she had become hypertensive. In fact, she had been drinking about six cups of liquorice tea per day. Whilst awaiting the results of her investigations for high blood pressure, she carried out some research herself. She found out liquorice does contribute to high blood pressure. This lady, upon becoming aware of this finding, immediately stopped using liquorice tea. The result? Her blood pressure improved spontaneously without any treatment.

One meta-analysis[29] pooled together eighteen studies involving liquorice. The researchers found that chronic ingestion of liquorice does significantly increase both systolic blood pressure and diastolic blood pressure. The keyword there is "chronic" use. By the way, chronic use refers to using the product over a medium to long term period. Occasional use will not produce the same effect. The mode of action is the active ingredient in liquorice which is glycyrrhizic acid or glycyrrhizin. The glycyrrhizic acid promotes renin activity which dovetails into the reduction of potassium levels in the blood through the kidneys. It does so by promoting aldosterone hormone activity[29].

You will recall we talked about the effect of high aldosterone levels previously in an earlier chapter. Liquorice raises your blood pressure by revving up aldosterone. Indeed, chronic use of liquorice is to be discouraged. Using it occasionally may be considered okay. But we have a problem. It is not entirely clear how much liquorice can be consumed safely by the general public.

The United Kingdom National Health Service website recommends eating less than 2 ounces of liquorice per day as a ballpark figure to go by[30]. Consuming more than that can potentially result in serious health problems such as hypertension and irregular heart rhythm especially if you are over 40. Indeed, my advice would be if you are somebody who is already hypertensive, steering clear of liquorice altogether won't be a bad idea after all.

Bitter Orange

Bitter orange is grown in the Middle East, South East Asia, East Africa and lately now being grown in California and Florida because of the favourable weather conditions in the two states. Bitter orange has been used in Chinese traditional medicine for centuries, for all sorts of ailments including heartburn, appetite suppression, boosting athletic performance, weight loss, constipation, nasal stuffiness, indigestion and nausea[31].

The active ingredient in bitter orange is synephrine. Synephrine has a chemical structural resemblance to ephedrine. If you remember, ephedrine use in weight loss products was banned by the FDA years ago because of its effect on blood pressure. So, it stands to reason that a product that has a chemical structure resembling that of ephedrine will have a similar effect on blood pressure or at least something close. This is the snag with bitter orange.

Let me draw your attention to this study[32] which was a small study but a well-designed one all the same. It involved fifteen young healthy adults who were randomised in this study. The keyword there is "healthy", meaning they did not have high blood pressure issues prior to being enlisted in the study. It was also a double-blinded placebo-controlled study. A double-blinded study is one where both the study participants and the researchers are unaware of which treatment or intervention the study participants are receiving until the study has ended. In this trial, the subjects were given Nature's Way bitter orange which contained 6% synephrine and a matching placebo with a one-week wash out. A wash out period is an intervention-free period which allows the body to completely rid itself of the effect of an earlier intervention before the second intervention is introduced. A wash out period prevents a "carry-over" effect from an earlier intervention or treatment making for more reliable result.

What they found was that the bitter orange significantly increased both the systolic and diastolic blood pressures and more importantly they found out that the effects lasted for up to five hours after a single dose of the bitter orange pill. Remember, these are healthy adults. And it's not just the effect on blood pressure alone that is the problem. In fact, there have been several case reports of people using products containing bitter orange, or its active ingredient synephrine, who have had heart attacks[33,34]. Fortunately, these individuals survived to tell the tale.

I mentioned this to serve as a warning. You should be on the lookout for products with synephrine in them. Pay special attention to weight loss products where they may sneak in synephrine as part of the formula. You must avoid them, at least for the purpose of controlling your blood pressure.

Weight Loss Products

There are two types of weight loss product: the ones you can buy over the counter and prescription-only weight loss medications. I have briefly touched on the over-the-counter weight loss products that are available in supermarkets and online e-commerce stores in the preceding section about bitter orange. The major task for anyone considering using these over-the-counter pills is identifying the individual ingredients that make up the formula and their possible side effects. Familiarity with all of the ingredients listed, and an awareness of the safety of each ingredient listed in the formula, is important. From our point of view, knowing that all the listed ingredients in a product's formula do not have the potential to cause elevated blood pressure is important.

This can be a problem, as millions of users do not have prerequisite knowledge of most ingredients. In the previous section, I talked about bitter orange, which may be listed as an ingredient in the formula of a weight loss product. I am willing to take a bet that millions of people on the planet are unaware that the active ingredient in bitter orange is synephrine. Knowing that synephrine is on a list of ingredients is one thing but being aware that synephrine elevates blood pressure is quite another. You have a scenario in which a product has bitter orange listed on the packet, meaning the manufacturer has complied with existing regulations. However, the user is totally unaware of one important side effect: the potential to raise the user's blood pressure.

The user of the product may now go to see his/her doctor and may wonder why a diagnosis of hypertension is being made. That is if the user is lucky enough to have symptoms in the first place, as hypertension is a largely asymptomatic disease in its early stages. If you do not have any symptoms, then you will be totally unaware that you are now a hypertensive patient. And, of course, target organ damage would be ongoing in the background; target organ damage that you are totally ignorant to. This is just one scenario where ignorance isn't bliss. Caffeine is another ingredient that these manufacturers tend to sneak into their formulas too. And extremely high doses of caffeine, I should add – much more caffeine than you would ordinarily consume in one cup of coffee. Be on the lookout if you are considering using any of these products. In my opinion, a lot of the weight loss products that are available over the counter are not worth the risk. Now, let us turn our attention to the prescription medications for weight loss.

The objective of prescription weight loss products is to stimulate satiety, and that dovetails into the reduction of hunger and reduction of food cravings. Ultimately what we are trying to achieve here is a reduction in overall energy intake daily[35]. More importantly, the use of weight loss prescription pills is supposed to be complementary to a diet plan. Prescription weight loss pills should not be a singular tool for weight reduction.

I had a short but interesting stint in a weight loss clinic some years back. The reason I did that job was because I wanted to "get inside the heads" of individuals with weight management problems. I was keen to learn about the psychological aspects of weight gain and weight loss. Indeed, I learnt a lot in that interesting time in my career. I got a lot of insight as to why people have problems managing their weight. That is a story for another day though.

While I worked at the clinic, the criteria we used at the time for prescribing medications for weight loss were:

a) BMI of ≥30 kg/m²
b) BMI of ≥27 kg/m² if that individual had associated weight-related problems like type 2 diabetes, osteoarthritis etc.

This guideline[36] bears a resemblance to the one that governed our use of pharmacological agents for the purpose of weight reduction at the time. I am not sure if the spine of the guideline has changed over the years, but I will doubt that very much. I do remember declining prescriptions for some patients whose BMI was just 27 kg/m² or over and who had no comorbidities (underlying medical problem). But they insisted on having the prescription. It usually took a lot of convincing to make the patient accept that it was possible for them to shed the desired amount of fat without any prescription intervention.

Part of the reason why we had these guidelines in place was because practically all the medications that we used had side effects. You could make that argument for practically all Big Pharma medications anyway, but I digress. One of the side effects was the potential for the user's blood pressure to become elevated whilst on the weight loss medication. But understandably some of the patients had difficulty seeing things from our point of view. If it is possible for you to shed your desired weight with diet and exercise, why put yourself through the process of using a pharmacological medication that has the potential to hand you hypertension as a gift?

Besides, weight loss from prescription pills (as with all other fat loss interventions) is not linear. Over the course of a year, the weight loss journey seen by most patients was something along the lines of - weight loss, weight regain, followed by further weight loss, followed by further regain, in that order. Such a sequence of events was very typical, and a pretty common scenario. The point here is that prescription weight loss medications are not the panacea for ultimate weight loss. So, what prescription pills are we talking about?

Four medications – phentermine, diethylpropion, phendimetrazine, and benzphetamine – have been in use for well over four decades. They have FDA approval too just in case you are wondering. These medications have a structural relationship to amphetamines and this chemical "zygosity" is particularly important physiologically. Of the four medications, the most popular in terms of prescription turnover is phentermine[37]. This drug is probably popular because it is cheaper and easy to use. Phentermine is also one of the most studied drugs on our list. Some studies[38,39] have shown a weight loss of between 5–10% in the first year of use. These kinds of published results bear resemblance to my experience at the weight loss centre. Remember, though, that weight loss is not a linear graph.

Lately, combination preparations, like phentermine and topiramate, are thought to yield better results[40], hence phentermine/topiramate and naltrexone/bupropion combinations have been given approval by the FDA, along with some newer agents: orlistat, lorcaserin and liraglutide[41]. It's important to remember that whilst the concept of drug combination therapy may be a good idea, it could also result in a multiplicity of side effects. It's just the name of the game – you won't always have it your way. It's important for both the doctor and the user to watch out for unpleasant side effects when using these new combination pills.

Regardless of whether single therapy or combination prescription pills are used, the anticipated picture is a weight reduction in the region of 5% in the first four months of use. Yes, most weight reduction on a new pill occurs during the honeymoon period. If the weight reduction on a particular prescription pill is not significant in the first four months, that medication will be discontinued, and consideration will be given to the use of another medication. The reason we did this was because of the side effects of these medications. Why continue with a medication that wasn't working well but had the potential to cause side effects? One of the side effects, of course, was elevated blood pressure. Other side effects included dry mouth, constipation, insomnia, and nervousness.

Because we were concerned with the effect of these medications on blood pressure, we ensured every patient's blood pressure was checked on every visit. If the blood pressure was elevated, the medication was discontinued straight away. Of course, we made sure the blood pressure was normal before commencing treatment. If the blood pressure was borderline elevated on the first visit, the medication was not started for obvious reasons. You will recall I mentioned earlier on that these medications have structural similarity to amphetamine. Amphetamine is a stimulant with negative impacts on blood pressure.

Ma Huang and Xenadrine

Ma huang is used in traditional Chinese medicine and has been around for centuries. But there is a problem with ma huang: it contains ephedrine, and ephedrine is banned because of its dangerous side effects. A particularly worrying side effect of ephedrine is its ability to raise blood pressure significantly with potentially fatal consequences on heart health. Over 200 episodes of heart attacks, strokes and 100 deaths had been reported to the FDA between 1993 and 2002 according to records obtained by the watchdog group called Public Citizen. Of course, we can easily link these problems to high blood pressure and the direct effect of ephedrine on the heart itself as it can make the heart beat extremely fast.

That isn't all. Ephedrine has psychiatric side effects too. There is the true story of an American lady who, after taking an ephedrine supplement in 1998, rammed her car into another car at 100 mph, killing two Canadian teenagers. She was tried in court and was unfortunately found not guilty by a British Columbian judge. Why did she get away with this? Well, because her lawyers argued she was not of sane mind at the time of the accident. Being under the influence of an ephedra supplement meant she was psychotic. The judge upheld the defence's argument and found the lady not guilty. The truth of the matter is the problems related to the use of ephedrine are too significant to allow the continued use of ephedrine in any preparations. But I do not think we are winning that battle just yet as you will see shortly with my quick research on the matter.

There is an argument that the way ephedrine is formulated in the West is the reason there are so many reported significant side effects. The Chinese argue that ephedrine should not be used in isolation as an ingredient; they posit that if ephedrine is combined with other ingredients, its side effects will be ameliorated. That argument may sound logical, but whether this is the reason the Chinese can use ma huang without these issues is debatable.

Now let me turn your attention to another popular ingredient – xenadrine. Is there any difference between ephedrine and xenadrine? Not really. If you remember in the spring of 2003, Steve Bechler of the Baltimore Orioles died following a collapse during a training session in the spring of that year. Steve Bechler had been using a product called Xenadrine RFA-1. The poor guy died at the tender age of 23 presumably using the product to boost his athletic performance. The medical examiner had no problems laying the cause of death on the footsteps of Xenadrine RFA-1. His widow sued the supplement manufacturer, and the matter was settled out of court. This incident led to a ban on all supplements containing ephedra alkaloids in February 2004 – or so you would think. I say this because from a quick look at an online marketplace and other independent websites, you will still find products containing ephedra, and others with xenadrine labels on them, being sold as we speak. The ban is not being enforced. The products are still very much around!

Here is something you should know. There is no difference between ephedra and xenadrine. They are the same. When I explored further, some of the products will have ma huang listed as opposed to ephedra (ephedrine) or xenadrine. Both the ephedra and the xenadrine come from the ma huang plant. Do not be fooled by their cryptic labelling – they are all the same. I do not blame people for getting sucked into using these potentially dangerous products for weight loss. The advertising pushes your emotional buttons to fall for the hype. For instance, one product talks about "the first of many dates" after losing the weight. Who doesn't want to go on as many dates as possible when they are looking for a partner? Another says, "Show your ex what he's missing". Ah, classic. Who wouldn't fall for a product that promises to get you "that body" – the one that will make your ex-partner regret his actions? You get the idea.

Another worrying trend I saw was how the supplement manufacturers stack up some of these ingredients. There was a weight loss supplement that had xenadrine, bitter orange and green coffee extract all stacked up together to achieve maximum effect. Of course, taking a product like this would send your endurance levels through the roof. You would work out all day if you wanted to and you would shed the fat – that much is true. But at what expense? Nervous jitters, an extremely fast heart rate, a thumping heart and raised blood pressure, all of which can lead to death. These ingredient combinations are potentially deadly. Take it from me. Ma huang, ephedra and xenadrine are bad news for your blood pressure. They are best avoided.

Over-the-Counter Cough and Cold Medications

The most used agents in cough and cold over-the-counter preparations are ephedrine, pseudoephedrine, phenylpropa-nolamine, and phenylephrine. Do these agents have an impact on blood pressure? The only reason I present you with this question is because the amounts used in cough and cold prepa-rations are less than you will find in standard prescription pills. Looking at the literature, the results are mixed. Also note-worthy is the fact that a lot of these studies have only produced weak evidence. We also do not have copious data on chronic use of these preparations. The average time these medications were used by participants in these studies is just four weeks[42] and, for the most part, that is about how long most users will consume these relief agents for.

The data available suggests that pseudoephedrine and phenylephrine may have the least effect on blood pressure in people who do not have high blood pressure[43]. It is important to remember that these medications stimulate the sympathetic nervous system. Anything that stimulates the sympathetic nervous system raises blood pressure just like the parasympathetic nervous system does the opposite – lowers it. Whilst pseudoephedrine and phenylephrine may appear safe in most people who do not have high blood pressure, care must be exercised by those who are hypertensive as the effect on them would be totally different. For instance, in this study[44] that looked at data from a stroke registry, pseudoephedrine was associated with strokes in 50% of the patients reviewed in the study. Several of the patients had pre-existing hypertension at the time the stroke occurred. Therein lies my cautionary note. Phenylpropanolamine and ephedrine are the worst of the agents. Phenylpropanolamine was implicated in the stroke cases in that study too. From the evidence available, it would be wise to avoid all cough and cold over-the-counter medications that have ephedrine and phenylpropanolamine in their ingredient list for safety reasons[45]. This is particularly important if you are someone who already has hypertension.

Anti-Migraine Medications

A couple of years ago, I was staring at the doors of half a century on this planet. Yes, little old me was approaching 50 at the time; an inevitable life event that will happen to billions of people lucky enough to hit the milestone. Remember, some don't make it that far in life through no fault of their own. I was one of the lucky ones. I had no idea how I had allowed all of that time to disappear on my watch without achieving many of the goals I had set myself. I believe age 50 is a watershed moment in one's life. Those who have gone through this phase in their lives know what I am talking about. If you are younger than 50, please enjoy the moment because time is one heck of an expensive currency – you heard it here first. Time is an *awfully* expensive currency. I needed to repeat that for emphasis. Anyway, out of the blue, I started having strange episodes of recurrent headaches. This happened for about five months. The headaches behaved exactly like migraine headaches. I had never had a migraine in the preceding 49 years of my life. So, this came to me as a not-so-pleasant surprise.

As it happens, I was able to treat the headaches with regular painkillers (acetaminophen) and a short course of nonsteroidal anti-inflammatory medications on each occasion. I try to avoid using nonsteroidal anti-inflammatory medications as much as possible, only taking them when absolutely necessary, like in this case, and for a very short duration. This is my attempt to protect my kidneys and prevent making my hypertension worse. This meant I was spared the next task of using triptans to deal with my migraine attacks. Another stroke of luck that I had at the time was that the headache episodes stopped after five months and have not returned ever since – thank goodness for that. It did make me wonder, though, why 50-year-old me at the time would start having migraines at such a late stage in life.

Migraine headaches are a common and potentially debilitating medical disorder. They are common enough to affect 12% of the US population[46]. The pathophysiology of the typical migraine is still not clear even now. The typical migraine headache affects one side of the brain, is of sudden onset and can be quite intense. As the science stands as we speak, we seem to think that there are some electrophysiological changes happening in the brain along with vascular changes. One possible explanation is that involving a complex spreading of a specific brain wave activity followed by suppression of brain activity[47]. This triggers a host of nerve and blood vessel functional events.

The blood vessel changes refer to vasodilatation which means the blood vessels relax and open up. The nerve at the base of the brain referred to as the trigeminal nerve is involved in this vasodilatation process.

The theory is that the trigeminal nerve releases some proteins called calcitonin gene-related peptides (CGRP). CGRP promotes relaxation of blood vessel walls which causes the vessels to relax and widen their capacity (vasodilatation)[48]. Because the trigeminal nerve is involved with sensation in the face as well as motor functions, including biting and chewing, you can see why migraine sufferers experience symptoms related to these aspects in addition to their headache. Most mild to moderate migraines will respond to a combination of nonsteroidal anti-inflammatory medications and regular analgesics like acetaminophen (aka Tylenol or Paracetamol), as happened in my case. If there is a poor response, however, then there is cause for using the next line of therapy – triptans. Triptans are usually reserved for moderate to severe migraines.

There are other therapies available for migraines like the ergotamines. What interests us here however as far as hypertension is concerned are the triptans. Vasodilatation as mentioned earlier on is one of the mechanisms involved in the pathophysiology of migraines. It therefore makes sense that if you are going to manage migraines successfully you may have to use a pharmacological agent that constricts the blood vessels. You essentially need to enact the opposite action to that which is causing the problem. Vasodilatation is one mechanism of migraines, and therefore it is necessary to administer medications that constrict the blood vessels (vasoconstrictors).

Triptans like sumatriptan, rizatriptan, almotriptan, zolmitriptan, naratriptan, eletriptan and frovatriptan do that job very well. Triptans perform this function through their action on two serotonin receptors – 5-HT1B and 5-HT1D. The two receptors are located on the smooth muscle cells on the walls of our blood vessels. Triptans are agonists (friends) to those two receptors. The problem for us, though, is that if you constrict the blood vessels, your blood pressure will rise. That is basic physiology. So, there is concern here as to whether triptans will raise blood pressure in normal people. I had a good look at the literature, and it does not look like the triptans have the potential to cause hypertension from the baseline of normality. It is possible that a user will have the blood pressure elevated but it is temporary without lasting damage. Migraine itself is a risk factor for stroke though[49]. So, using an agent that constricts blood vessels puts the user at risk of developing a stroke. As stated earlier, the evidence does suggest that triptan use may not be a cause of hypertension in normotensive individuals.

But the picture in people with high blood pressure is different. Triptans should be used with caution in individuals who already have pre-existing hypertension especially if poorly controlled. Caution should also be exercised when using triptans in people with vascular disease, poorly controlled diabetes, or hemiplegic migraine because of the real risk of causing a stroke[50]. So, while triptans may not be a true cause of hypertension in individuals with normal blood pressure, they may be a nuisance in people who are already hypertensive.

Antidepressants

There are many antidepressants available on the market. The very first class of antidepressants marketed are the monoamine oxidase inhibitors. These were in use for many years but became less popular due to concerns regarding toxicity and lesser efficacy compared to the next generation of antidepressants: tricyclic antidepressants[51]. There has been a resurgence of some of these medications recently, mainly because we have a better understanding of how some of them work. Some are now being used for treatment of non-endogenous depressive and anxiety syndromes, which are also described as "atypical depression" in layman's terms.

Newer technologies available now mean that some of the newer monoamine oxidase inhibitors can be administered through the skin. These are called transdermal preparations, and they are available as options for managing patients with unipolar, bipolar, atypical, and treatment-resistant depression[52].

The next group of medications that are used in depression are those we refer to as tricyclic antidepressants. These medications appear to have complex interactions with different tissues in the human body, therefore the use of these medications on patients suffering from depression must be individualised. Their complex interactions mean that doctors are usually very careful when treating depressed patients with these tricyclic antidepressants especially in patients who have underlying cardiovascular diseases like high blood pressure. Care is also exercised in patients who have glaucoma and those who tend to suffer from urinary retention[53].

Whilst we are on the subject of managing mental health problems, let me just quickly touch on another condition that has a bearing on blood pressure. I am referring to adult attention deficit hyperactivity disorder (ADHD). ADHD is a common mental health problem with accompanying high disability and frequent co-morbidity. The most common medications used to manage ADHD are methylphenidate and atomoxetine. However, their success rate is only good in the short to medium term. The fact that there is poor response to these two medications in the long term means alternative pharmacological agents have to be sought for the benefit of these patients. The alternative compounds are mainly the amphetamines which have proven efficacy. The problem with the amphetamines, however, is the fact they have the propensity to increase blood pressure. This is a problem that limits their use in the long term, and this also makes them unsuitable for use by patients who have hypertension[54]. If you are on amphetamine-related medication and you are struggling to have your blood pressure under control, your doctor may want to review that prescription.

Now, let's talk about a somewhat innocent group of medications that arguably one in five adults in the industrialised world are using today. These medications have a bearing on blood pressure, and they are called selective serotonin reuptake inhibitors (SSRIs). SSRIs are by far one of the most popular group of medications prescribed by doctors today, especially in the developed world. They work by inhibiting (reducing) serotonin reuptake within the nervous system, which means serotonin accumulates and is readily available. SSRI pills are so widely used that they are as popular as blood pressure medications. In fact, for Big Pharma, SSRIs are an evergreen cash cow. Thanks to the world we live in today which makes mental health problems a skyrocketing phenomenon. It is estimated that 792 million people suffer from one mental health problem or the other globally[55]. That is one in ten people. I still think the incidence is much higher than that as there is a lot of under-reporting. The incidence is certainly higher in industrialised nations. Of course, anxiety and depression are high up on the list. SSRIs are just what the doctor ordered. This SSRI popularity does come at a price though. The price being side effects. One of those side effects is high blood pressure. What surprised me when I was looking at the literature regarding the association between SSRI medications and hypertension was that the SSRIs can cause hypertension in younger people using the medications too.

One observational study[56] that followed up 11,183 individuals over a period of fourteen years showed this association between the use of antidepressants and hypertension. The antidepressant group of medications with the most impact on blood pressure were SSRIs. The participants in this study were followed up from adolescence and, by the time they were 29, the prevalence of hypertension amongst the antidepressant users was 20% even after accounting for depressive symptomatology and behavioural factors. There was an association with the use of non-SSRI medications too, but SSRIs were more impactful on blood pressure. Negative impact, that is.

There is a concept in medicine called pharmacovigilance. It is the process of monitoring adverse effects of medications. Pharmacovigilance is a continuous dynamic process. Pharmacovigilance is a never-ending process. When medications are monitored on a continuous basis for decades, some adverse effects may become apparent with time. One example that springs to mind is Reye's syndrome which became apparent with the use of aspirin. And this association between aspirin and Reye's syndrome was the direct result of reporting and analysing of the side effects plugged into the vigilance database. Aspirin has had an easy ride with pharmacovigilance, especially considering the consequences for some other medications, which have suffered a worse fate.

Rofecoxib (Vioxx) was approved in 1999. The drug manufacturer did not list any cardiovascular side effects when licensing was applied for. When Vioxx was unleashed eighteen months later onto the market, reports of serious cardiovascular events began to emerge. But it was a trial for using Vioxx for polyp prevention that gave the game away. Participants in the trial were noted to be having episodes of heart attacks and strokes[57]. The FDA had seen enough. Vioxx was withdrawn from the market forthwith in 2004. That is barely five years of being on the market.

Another example is cisapride. This drug was approved for gastroesophageal reflux disease (GERD). Cisapride enjoyed a wild ride with gastroenterologists who were really impressed with its performance. That was until reports of significant cardiovascular side effects and even deaths associated with this "wonderful" drug started to surface from the depths of the blue sea of GERD relief. Eighty deaths were linked to cisapride use. Cisapride swallowed its pride in 2000 and was sunk swiftly never to be seen again[58].

One way of looking at pharmacovigilance is to see it as post-marketing surveillance. Pharmacovigilance is designed to protect the public from collateral harm that these medications may possess. Harm that may not be obvious in the drug trial phases before drug approval by regulatory authorities. One hopes Big Pharma is not playing a "cat and mouse" game with regulatory authorities. Not disclosing all there is to know when applying for drug approval. That would be a silly thing to do as these secrets will rear their ugly heads over time.

Why am I talking about pharmacovigilance here? Well, it is because pharmacovigilance has demonstrated a rather clear association between the SSRIs and hypertension. Reports emerging from the World Health Organisation pharmacovigilance database and the French pharmacovigilance database have shown links between these SSRIs and high blood pressure[59]. Women seem to be affected more than men. The mean age for this hypertension complication from SSRI use is the mid-50s[59]. The guiltiest SSRIs are sertraline and paroxetine. But fluoxetine, citalopram, escitalopram and fluvoxamine aren't exactly angels in this affair. They are equally guilty. Only a little less than sertraline and paroxetine. I suppose the reason these medications are still on the market is that these side effects which, of course, includes high blood pressure are not seen as life threatening enough by regulatory authorities to justify a complete ban and withdrawal from the market.

The Combined Oral Contraceptive Pill

These seemingly innocent pills we use for family planning have the potential to cause hypertension. How soon after using the pill can a woman develop high blood pressure? Well, the hypertension effects can begin as early as six months. But hypertension is more likely to occur with longer use and may not happen until six years later[60]. As for how often hypertension can occur in combined oral contraceptive pill users, epidemiological studies put the incidence at 5%[61]. In the US, where there is a sizeable population of Latino women, the figure is higher.

When a cohort of Latino women in El Paso who cross the US-Mexico border to obtain contraceptive pills over the counter were studied, the incidence of hypertension in combined oral contraceptive pill users was 10.5%[62]. The good news is that most of the women who develop high blood pressure would have a mild form of the disease. The hypertension will equally resolve upon stopping the pill. A few cases of severe hypertension have been reported in the scientific literature though[63]. As for which women are likely to develop hypertension on the combined pill, the risk of developing hypertension rises in women who had high blood pressure during a pregnancy, those who smoke, those who are overweight with a BMI of 30 and over, those with a family history of hypertension and women over 35 years of age.

It behoves on doctors to screen women who are at risk of hypertension and not prescribe them the pill. But women are capable of self-screening themselves when provided with the right tool. The right tool could be as simple as a medical checklist provided to women. This study[64] in El Paso involving 1271 women proved this simple checklist tool can be just as effective as a doctor's screening. It just goes to show that if you empower health care users, they can deliver results when provided with appropriate tools.

Prescription

Be careful what over-the-counter pills you get yourself for whatever reason you want them. There are high blood pressure side effects lurking around a lot of these over-the-counter supplements.

Weight loss supplements in particular do pack a punch with high blood pressure side effects. Even the prescription weight management pills, although your doctor should take care of the associated risks in prescription pills. But you have sole responsibility for what happens with over-the-counter supplements.

Look out for ingredients like bitter orange, synephrine, ephedra, caffeine, ma huang, xenadrine etc. If you see any of those in the list of ingredients, do not use that supplement. Avoid using liquorice-containing products of any kind. At least in the medium to long term anyway.

Be careful with antidepressants and that includes over-the-counter St John's Wort. Between you and your doctor, you should be mindful of your use of prescription antidepressants, stimulants for ADHD, prescription nonsteroidal anti-inflammatory and the cox-2 inhibitor medications etc. These prescription medications are potential fault lines for development of hypertension and poor control of your blood pressure. They must be substituted if these medications make themselves a nuisance to your blood pressure control efforts.

CHAPTER 4

The Caffeine Effect

I decided to dedicate a whole chapter to caffeine in this book because caffeine is worth it. And you will find out why when you are done with this chapter. The fact that caffeine is a buzzword, and that caffeine gives us a buzz when consumed is neither news to your ears nor is it arguable in the twenty-first century. Caffeine is undoubtedly the most consumed pharmacologically active agent worldwide. The average intake of caffeine in the US stands at 200–300 mg per day in three-quarters of adults[65].

Thomas Jefferson once said, "Coffee – the favourite drink of the civilised world."

The coffee industry is huge. It is a multibillion-dollar industry annually, and it continues to grow. Brazil, Vietnam, and Columbia, the three biggest producers of coffee in that order as of 2019, are not complaining about the popularity of this seemingly innocent bean[66]. There's money to be made from coffee and they are going for it. And why not? If you have weather that favours the growth of the bean and you have established export logistics and infrastructure in place, then go for it. We can't seem to get enough of the coffee bean.

But how was coffee discovered and how did we come to fall in love with coffee? Let's dive a little bit into the history of coffee and how it became such a huge export commodity, as well as a must-have "thing" in one form or another to brighten our day. As Brazil tops the charts in coffee production today, you would think that coffee's origins would be traceable back to Brazil, wouldn't you? You would be wrong if you thought that!

Where did it all start then?

Legend has it coffee had its origin in the plains and highlands of Ethiopia in the kingdom of Sheba. A gentleman named Kaldi was a goat farmer. Kaldi noticed something peculiar about his goats' attitude and behaviour. His goats were attracted to some red berries from a particular tree. Every time the goats fed on these berries, they had awesome energy. The goats were unusually excited. They jumped around on their hind legs, bleating louder than normal.

He passed his observation on to a monk, who was curious enough to try these berries out for himself, but only after he overcame his initial suspicion. The monk initially threw these strange berries away, but they accidentally landed in a fire. That singular act of accidentally casting the berries into a fire turned out to be serendipitous. The aroma from roasted coffee, as you probably know, is plain gorgeous. It was then, and it still is now. The beautiful aroma from the berries being burnt made him change his mind.

The monk retrieved the berries and soaked them in hot water to put out the fire. He decided on a whim to drink the flavoured water from these berries. The monk could not believe how alert he was during his prayer and other spiritual devotions. Soon, other monks participated in this red berry experiment, and they had a similar result. "Awesome discovery", they told themselves. They couldn't get enough of these berries.

The news of these wonderful berries known as *bunn* spread to the Arabian Peninsula. They got hold of the plant, cultivated it and it soon became a very nice drink to have. Consumers found the little highs from having the bean desirable.

Coffee houses sprang up in Persia, Yemen, Turkey, Syria, Egypt, and other North African habitats. These houses were known as *qahveh khaneh*. These coffee houses became a social hub for a lot of communities. Religion helped the spread of coffee beyond the Middle East too. Pilgrims visiting Mecca annually meant pilgrims had a taste of what was called "wine of Araby"[67]. They liked it and, of course, took some coffee seeds back home with them. Part of the appeal to the Islamic world was that the "wine of Araby" was a good substitute for real wine. More importantly, coffee was seen as a good fasting tool; it helped Muslims fast during the daytime and had the potential to keep them awake at night during the period of Ramadan[68].

The genie was now out of the bottle. Coffee's arrival in Europe was not met with universal approval though. Some hated the drink especially in Venice in 1615 where one clergy described coffee as "the bitter invention of Satan"[67]. Pope Clement VIII got involved in the coffee drama, or should we call it the "black drink drama"? He tasted it. Loved it. And gave it a papal seal of approval. End of squabble. If the Pope said it was good, then it was good. No arguments.

From the Vatican, the coffee migration was heading west. It moved across to England, Austria, France, Germany, and Holland. Lots of coffee houses sprouted all over England by the mid-seventeenth century. These coffee houses became business hubs in England. Deals were discussed and struck in these coffee houses. The same legend has it that Lloyd's of London was a product of such business meetings in Edward Lloyd's Coffee House. Across the pond, coffee arrival there in the New World, as it was then called (now the US), did not enjoy an easy ride. Americans favored tea over this new black bitter drink.

That was until King George III slammed a huge tax on tea to give the East India Company (the biggest tea exporter to the British colonies) an unfair market competitive advantage. This was the Tea Act of 1773. This Act caused a mutiny against the British government in 1773, referred to as the Boston Tea Party[69]. The increased taxation forced Americans to rethink their tea consumption. As fate would have it, the resistance to the Tea Act became the catalyst for the American Revolution that led to her independence from Great Britain.

An alternative to tea was sought at the time because of the tea boycott. Coffee presented itself. This tea substitute from then on gradually snuck into American culture quietly and has never left. If anything, coffee grew deeper roots in the consumption habits of Americans. In fact, John Adams considered tea drinking as an unpatriotic act post-American revolution. Coffee became the preferred hot drink in America. Where there is profit to be made, you can expect self-preservation and protectionism. Coffee's popularity soared across the globe, so did competition to cultivate and market it. Some governments tried and failed to cultivate it. Others succeeded. The weather had to be right.

Let's fast forward to how Brazil became the biggest producer of coffee. We can trace this to the theory that being blessed with charisma and ravishing physical looks may lead to good fortune. Thank your parents if their union gave you not just the gift of life but looks to die for. Francisco de Mello Palheta was one of these lucky folks – he was easy on the eye. In 1727, Francisco had been sent on an ambassadorial errand to French Guiana to get some coffee seedlings, but sources claim the French were reluctant to part with them. Not very many people are willing to share their cash cow, and you could argue that this is human nature. Others will disagree, saying generosity is a virtue.

However, the wife of the French governor of French Guiana had other ideas, regardless of how her husband felt. When you like someone, you will bend over backwards to please that person, and Mrs Governor had a crush on Francisco. She had a cunning plan to please the man she admired. She presented Francisco with a bouquet of flowers with coffee seeds buried inside. Those seeds represent the humble beginnings of this multibillion-dollar coffee industry that we've come to know and love. Because Francisco de Mello Palheta, on arrival back home in Brazil, planted the gifted coffee seeds in the northeastern territory of Brazil. The seeds grew, thrived, and, of course, more were cultivated. Brazilian soil was particularly good for the coffee plant. Such that by 1770 the coffee plantation adventure had spread south of the country and by 1830, Brazil was producing 30% of the world's coffee.

Okay, let's get back to the impact of coffee on blood pressure. One of the hottest controversies in the medical and nutraceutical world is the effect of coffee – or should I say caffeine – on the cardiovascular system. More specifically, the effect of caffeine on blood pressure. The debate around coffee is just below that of diet wars in terms of ranking. You know the one: fat versus carbs. Doesn't the fat versus carbs debate just drive you mad? Or make you yawn…

Let's not forget that coffee and other caffeinated products, including tea and chocolate, constitute a multibillion-dollar industry. When there are vested interests and money to be made, then expect a push-back if the image of caffeine is being trashed publicly. Some livelihoods depend on our continued interest and relentless addiction to coffee. When you dive into the medical literature, prepare to have a fabulous time with conflicting research findings. What is clear from the research, though, is that coffee – or indeed caffeine – does have some health benefits. At the same time, however, caffeine does have an impact on blood pressure, most of which is negative. I will explain the nature of this impact in a minute.

Let us start with the positives first. I believe some researchers are so captivated by the benefits of caffeine or coffee that they cannot accept the negative aspects of caffeine can and do have clinical significance. Truth be told, coffee does contain good antioxidants. Antioxidants that your body needs. Antioxidants like chlorogenic acid and other compounds like trigonelline, ferulic acid, caffeic acid, and n-coumaric acid. The process of roasting also leads to the release of compounds like melanoidins. Melanoidins are brown pigments induced by the process of roasting. Melanoidins are antioxidants too[70].

All coffee products, however, are not created equal. Where the coffee plant is grown influences the antioxidant content within it. Arabica coffee, grown and harvested in Mexico and India, has been shown to have higher polyphenols when compared to coffee cultivated in China, for instance. The extraction process also plays a role in how much chlorogenic acid and other beneficial compounds are left in the final product[71]. So, whilst we might celebrate the friendly offers of the antioxidants in our coffee, it may be a good idea to take a pause and reflect on how much goodness there *really* is in each individual coffee product we purchase. What I mean is that the antioxidant benefits of coffee are not always guaranteed in all coffee products.

The belief in some quarters in the benefits of coffee is so strong that one condensed review of epidemiological evidence went as far as suggesting a 15% reduction in cardiovascular disease when one habitually consumes three to five cups of coffee a day[72]. This review also says that drinking one to five cups a day is associated with a lower risk of death compared to drinking none. And what did this review say about coffee consumption in hypertensive individuals? The reviewers concluded that coffee consumption in large doses should be avoided in those with uncontrolled hypertension.

What about those with controlled high blood pressure? The researchers concluded that coffee consumption is probably safe in those with controlled hypertension. Note that they qualified their conclusion with the word "probably" – something tells me they are hedging their bets with that review.

Now let's look at the speed at which coffee is broken down when consumed. At play here will be genetics. You don't have any control here, folks. Unfortunately, your genes do. Your genes decide how quickly or slowly you metabolize your coffee. And where does this breakdown of caffeine begin? The liver, of course. Where else? The liver is the factory for the metabolism of most of the things we eat and drink, including drugs. Remember that caffeine is a drug. We have one enzyme to thank for this: cytochrome P450 1A2. It's a liver enzyme that has the job of breaking down the caffeine in our coffee, tea, or chocolate. The first byproduct of caffeine breakdown in the liver by cytochrome P450 1A2 is paraxanthine. By the way, how active this cytochrome P450 1A2 liver enzyme is wholly dependent on your age, smoking habit, gender and, of course, genetics. And by genetics, I am referring to a gene called CYP1A2.

If you have two copies of the gene P450 1A2 (CYP1A2), you are one of the lucky ones. You will be a fast caffeine metabolizer, meaning you can get rid of the caffeine in your coffee and other caffeinated products quickly. In contrast, if you have one copy of the gene, you are a carrier. Carriers are slow caffeine metabolizers. If you are a slow caffeine metabolizer, you'll have the caffeine hanging around your body a lot longer compared to a fast metabolizer. Sorry about that. I am one of you – a slow metabolizer. You might find some solace in that. Okay, maybe not. If you are keen to find out whether you are a slow metabolizer or a fast metabolizer, you can order genetic testing from one of the companies offering the service online. I won't name any one company here, at risk of promoting one over the other inadvertently. Do your own search online. And just go with any one of them that looks trustworthy.

Anyway, is it possible that people who have the gene for abnormal metabolism of coffee – the functional variant of P450 1A2 (CYP1A2) – are more at risk of cardiovascular disease with habitual coffee consumption? I am referring here to the "carriers" I mentioned earlier. A prospective analysis of 347,077 people did not find an association between carriers of the gene and cardiovascular risk with regular consumption. Do remember that carriers are slow metabolizers. However, a modest increase in cardiovascular risk with heavy coffee consumption in slow metabolizers was found in that study[73]. So, there was a small price to pay for heavy consumption if coffee hung around your body for longer if you drank more.

Interestingly, another study from Costa Rica that looked at 2,014 cases of non-fatal heart attacks says something totally different. They matched the 2,014 heart attack cases with an equal number of population-based controls. The researchers matched heart attack cases for age, sex, and area of residence. Additionally, they performed the genotype of the individuals in the study, looking for pairing of the P450 1A2 (CYP1A2) gene. So, what did the Costa Rican researchers find? The results are in direct contrast to the first study I mentioned. They found drinking four cups of coffee or more per day puts you at 1.5 times higher risk of non-fatal heart attacks if you are a male slow metabolizer. If you are a female slow metabolizer, your risk of non-fatal heart attack was 2.8 times higher. These results are in comparison to those who drank one cup of coffee or less per day[74].

For me, the findings in the second study make more sense. Slow metabolizers tend to have more issues with coffee and caffeine consumption especially if they typically drink more than one cup a day. In contrast, the caffeine is quickly dealt with by the liver and ushered out of the body at a faster rate in fast metabolizer individuals even when they consume more. If you are a slow metabolizer, however, the same logic dictates that you will have more of the caffeine hanging around your body much longer compared to a fast metabolizer. This means you are more likely to have side effects, as each subsequent cup of coffee you drink increases the circulating levels of caffeine in your blood; call it a cumulative effect if you like. The cardiovascular effects will therefore be more pronounced.

How about the direct effect of caffeine on blood pressure? Like I said earlier, you could have a lot of fun examining the literature on caffeine or coffee on blood pressure. Lots of fun and you will find yourself neck-deep in the avalanche of studies about. For the sake of being succinct, I have taken one meta-analysis[75] whose objective was to "summarize the evidence on the acute and longer-term effects of caffeine and coffee intake on BP and on the association between habitual coffee consumption and risk of cardiovascular disease in hypertensive individuals".

In this meta-analysis, they found consumption of 200–300 mg of caffeine resulted in a rise of the systolic blood pressure (the top number) of an average of 8.1 units and 5.7 mmHg rise in diastolic blood pressure (the bottom number). That rise might not look like much but if you put it into real life BP readings, it might make more sense. For instance, an initial blood pressure reading of 145/95 mmHg now becomes 153/100 mmHg or higher in real terms after drinking coffee. The review also found that the effect lasted for ≥ three hours. Their findings also suggest habitual consumption of caffeine does not lead to hypertension or increased cardiovascular complications. So, it might not lead to hypertension as a disease entity, but it will make your attempts at controlling your blood pressure more challenging.

Does consumption of coffee elevate your blood pressure at work or in a stressed environment? We drink a lot of coffee at work, don't we? So, it is nice to know what happens to our blood pressure when we drink cup after cup over the official eight hours of being in the office. This study[76] carried out on healthy volunteers tells us coffee at work does have an impact on our BP. It was a double-blind crossover study using caffeinated versus decaffeinated coffee. Blood pressure was monitored using an ambulatory blood pressure monitoring technique. What the researchers found in the study was that both the top blood pressure reading (systolic) and the bottom reading (diastolic) were raised on the days the study participants consumed caffeinated coffee.

What about when the subjects were subjected to mental arithmetic stress on either caffeinated coffee or decaffeinated coffee? Not surprisingly, the blood pressure readings were even higher on caffeine days when subjected to the stress of doing some mental arithmetic[76]. Never mind that these were healthy volunteers and not hypertensive individuals. What we can learn from this piece of research is that consumption of caffeine exaggerates your blood pressure response when under mental stress. This is in comparison to what happens when not under the influence of caffeine, even if you are not hypertensive. If that is the sort of cardiovascular response normotensive folks (i.e. those who do not have high BP) experience when stress and caffeine are combined, what would happen in those of us with hypertension? Well, it is not hard to imagine that the blood pressure elevation in hypertensive individuals who consume coffee at work would be predictably higher. This is particularly so when there is a demand on mental capabilities.

That is not all. The effect of caffeine consumption when under stress goes beyond the blood pressure increase. It affects the function of the left side of your heart too. The larger chamber on the left side of the heart (the left ventricle) was shown to do harder work in stressful caffeinated scenarios in another study[77]. The additive combination of stress and caffeine was enough to push the blood pressure of the participants of this second study into the hypertensive zone. These participants in the second study were also healthy, non-hypertensive individuals.

I want to briefly talk about one more study. Remember I did say you could get buried in caffeine studies if you really want to get nerdy with it. I did pay a bit of attention to this next study mainly because of the study design and the fact that the researchers had previously done quite some work on caffeine and blood pressure matters. What the researchers did was give caffeine to different groups of people. The groups recruited into the study were people with very normal blood pressure, those with normal blood pressure, those with high normal blood pressure, those with stage 1 hypertension and those with established hypertension[78]. They pooled the participants into those individual groups based on the Sixth Report of the Joint National Committee on Prevention, Detection, Evaluation, and Treatment of High Blood Pressure (JNC VI) hypertension definition[79].

The result of that research was a rise in both the systolic blood pressure (top reading) and the diastolic BP (bottom number) in all groups. However, there was a graduated elevation of blood pressure in the different groups. Meaning the higher your pre-caffeine BP was, the more elevated your post-caffeine BP reading was too. It was a linear response. In fact, those who had established hypertension had 1.5 times higher rise in both systolic and diastolic BP than those in the very normal BP group. What this piece of research is telling us is people with high blood pressure have a differential sensitivity to caffeine compared to the lucky folks without hypertension.

So, why does caffeine cause a blood pressure elevation? The truth of the matter is that caffeine is a drug: a vasoactive drug, a pharmacologically active drug. It may not be a prescription medication, but it is a drug all the same. Caffeine has a pressor effect on the vascular tree and increases the tone of the walls of our arteries. Anything that increases the tone of our arteries makes the arteries stiffer. A stiff artery will have a higher blood pressure reading. That's the first thing you need to know about caffeine.

The next thing you should know is that caffeine is attracted to a chemical receptor in the body called the adenosine receptor. This is the receptor – as the name implies – that gladly allows adenosine to perch upon it. Adenosine is what makes us feel tired, and not only gives you a feeling of fatigue, but also makes you feel sleepy. Adenosine is the substance that runs down our batteries every day. If you can find something that stops adenosine from doing its job, then you are in for a wild ride. Caffeine does that job perfectly. Caffeine is an adenosine blocker. If you block adenosine from perching on its receptors in the brain, you recharge your batteries albeit temporarily. That's how your coffee gives you the kick and the buzz after drinking it. Caffeine sits on the receptors for adenosine, more specifically the A1 and A2A adenosine receptors in the brain.

Adenosine is a nerve chemical that is produced from the minute we wake up and gradually builds up, reaching a crescendo at bedtime. When the adenosine receptors are taken up in the brain and the rest of the nervous system by caffeine, adenosine cannot attach itself. This displacement of adenosine from its parent receptors means adenosine is unable do its job effectively. The caffeine squatting on those adenosine receptors fires up the nerve cells. So, whereas adenosine slows down the nerve cell, the attached caffeine does the opposite. Caffeine gives the nerve cells some oomph. That's why you feel fired up after a cup of your coffee or caffeinated tea.

One other job that adenosine does is widen your blood vessels especially the blood vessels in the brain. The idea is to perfuse your brain with plenty of oxygen and nutrients when you are asleep. Caffeine does the exact opposite. Once the caffeine metabolites are perched on the adenosine receptors, they constrict the blood vessels. For this reason, caffeine is used for the treatment of the types of headaches we class as vascular headaches. For instance, the tablet Anacin contains aspirin and caffeine in its formula. Other headache medications with caffeine in them include Excedrin, Midol, Migranal and Fioricet. The drug manufacturers exploit this peculiar adenosine-blocking effect of caffeine that causes constriction of blood vessels, particularly the arteries. If you constrict blood vessels, blood pressure will rise representing an indirect mechanism through which caffeine may raise your blood pressure.

I will skip over the effect of caffeine on the A2A adenosine receptors but suffice to say that the A2A receptor blockade caused by caffeine results in the release of dopamine. That dopamine release is the reason you get the "feel good factor" when you consume coffee and other caffeinated products. Ever had someone advise you to have chocolate when your mood is somewhat on the low side? Those moments when you are feeling blue for no obvious reason. That's the source of that piece of advice; chocolate contains caffeine. Consuming chocolate will potentially lead to dopamine release and may make you feel better.

Next fact about caffeine effect is what caffeine does to the hormones in the body. Let us start with the hormone, cortisol. This is our stress hormone. Does caffeine affect our cortisol levels? The answer is yes, caffeine does influence our cortisol levels. And caffeine exerts its influence on cortisol by going direct to the higher centers – the brain. This piece of research[80] tested forty-seven healthy volunteers at rest for the effect of caffeine on cortisol. It was a double-blind placebo-controlled crossover study. The researchers found a rise in cortisol levels from one hour to two hours post-caffeine consumption. The peak rise of cortisol was at sixty minutes.

Not only that, but the researchers also tested whether the trigger was coming from the pituitary gland or not. One way of doing that is to test for blood levels of the cortisol activator hormone called adrenocorticotrophic hormone (ACTH) when caffeine is consumed. They did exactly that. They found the adrenocorticotrophic hormone to be elevated in tandem with the cortisol. Peak increase for the adrenocorticotrophic hormone was also found to be at sixty minutes too relative to placebo. The adrenocorticotrophic hormone is the hormone that triggers the release of cortisol from the adrenal glands. The adrenocorticotrophic hormone is produced in the pituitary gland in the brain. Caffeine influences this adrenocorticotrophic hormone too by stimulating its release from the pituitary even at rest. Once adrenocorticotrophic hormone release is stimulated from the pituitary, cortisol release is activated in the adrenals.

Is it possible to develop a tolerance to the cortisol-stimulating effects of caffeine if one is a regular caffeine consumer? There does appear to be some level of tolerance that develops in the habitual consumer, in that less cortisol is released over time. Before you go celebrating this cortisol plateau, however, there is research evidence to suggest that the desensitisation is not absolute[81].

Yes, it is true that cortisol release tolerance occurs in habitual caffeine users, but such tolerance is partial. The same research[81] found statistically significant elevations of cortisol during the afternoon hours with habitual caffeine consumption, even in healthy consumers. Tolerance effects occur mainly in the morning, so there is tolerance, but it is partial. When we are subjected to mental stress, the effect of caffeine on cortisol becomes exaggerated which is not surprising[82].

What about the effect of caffeine on adrenaline and nor-adrenaline? These are the other two stress hormones that are affected by caffeine in addition to cortisol. Much of the adren-aline we make comes from the adrenal glands. But the sister hormone, noradrenaline, is produced mainly from the sympa-thetic nervous system. You will be surprised to learn that only 10% of the noradrenaline comes from the adrenal gland. The other 90% is produced outside of the adrenal glands – periph-eral release. Caffeine does have a direct effect on target organs too[83]. The story of caffeine effect on adrenaline and noradrena-line is a direct effect on the adrenal glands and the sympathetic nervous system. Thus, the quantities of adrenaline and nor-adrenaline in blood circulation are elevated when we have had our lovely cup of coffee. Higher levels of both hormones are equally released when stress and caffeine are working together in tandem.

Something I would like you to know is that there is always a low level of noradrenaline activity buzzing around our body twenty-four hours a day. That low level threshold is maintained until we are subjected to stress of any type. Physical stress, mental or emotional stress will cause a breakthrough above that threshold. Caffeine consumption causes a breakthrough above the threshold too. Adrenaline is released at the same time as noradrenaline from the adrenal glands. The release is usually a sudden burst in readiness for fight or flight. Truth be told, caffeine revs up the sympathetic nervous system without doubt. How quickly and how large the magnitude of the rev-ving up will vary between individuals.

One important point to remember is this: most individu-als with primary hypertension (essential hypertension) have a high resting sympathetic tone. When your basal sympathetic tone is already relatively high, it only takes a little stimulus to move through the gears up very quickly. So, zero to sixty in four seconds or less like a sports car accelerating off on a racing track. This translates to blood pressure that is extremely sensitive to any sympathetic stimulation, because your resting sympathetic tone is already relatively high compared to an individual without high blood pressure. Caffeine is a substance that stimulates the sympathetic nervous system, and we can safely say that it is an agent ready to perform a task with that job description anytime you drink a mug of coffee.

I have dissected the effect of caffeine on blood pressure and the mechanisms through which caffeine exerts its influence accordingly. But do we have outliers? Yes, we do. We have outliers who respond just a little differently to the caffeine norm. For instance, there is a colleague of mine (a medical doctor too) who could be best described as a coffee addict. I do worry about her and her level of coffee consumption, but she reassures me that all is well with her.

She tells me her blood pressure is fine. She is in the sixth decade of her life, but she reports having good blood pressure readings. I have to say I haven't really confirmed her claim, but I want to believe her as she has no valid reason to lie to me. Okay, there is. If anything, to get me off her back. She is a lady who wakes up at 3 o'clock in the morning, heads downstairs and makes herself a cup of coffee. Yes, you read that right. She wakes up in the middle of the night to have coffee and goes back to bed after her ungodly hour coffee fix. If that's not addiction, then I don't know what is. The point I am making here is there are individuals who will respond just a little differently when they consume coffee or any other caffeinated drink for that matter.

Why is that? Well, we are all different, aren't we? You remember I talked about the slow metabolizers and the fast metabolizers. Those who are blessed with a paired up P450 1A2 (CYP1A2) gene are fast metabolizers. It is possible that these lucky folks break down their caffeine so fast, it doesn't have enough time to exert any untoward cardiovascular effect. So long as the kidneys are functioning well to flush out the breakdown products quickly too, my theory on this may well be true.

A second reason is that coffee and most other products containing caffeine have antioxidants in them as part of their natural constitution. Antioxidants have innate vessel relaxing effect on arteries. So, we have a situation here where there are two opposing effects: the caffeine's artery constricting effect and an opposing antioxidant vessel relaxing effect, all within the same product. I have thought about the different effects of caffeine on different people extensively.

My conclusion is that the question of whether a caffeinated product will cause a rise in your blood pressure or, contrastingly have a blood pressure lowering effect will wholly depend on which of those two forces wins the fight. If the dominant force is the vessel constricting influence, then a rise in blood pressure is to be expected. Conversely, if the antioxidant effect dominates, then a neutral effect or a blood pressure lowering effect will be the result. Another factor is the product's primary source. I know from experience that caffeine from cocoa beans seems to have a weak effect on blood pressure, thereby allowing the flavanols in cocoa beans to dominate. Hence cacao powder is one product I recommend for blood pressure reduction. I will touch on this in greater detail when the discussion centres on blood pressure self-management in the later segments of this book. Caffeine from coffee beans on the other hand possesses a more potent blood pressure hiking effect.

There is also age to consider. As we get older, our arteries stiffen up unless, of course, one has lived a relatively healthy life. On the typical Western diet, stiffer arteries are to be expected. When the vessel constrictive effects of caffeine meet an artery that is already stiff, then a rise in blood pressure is not unusual. Likewise, the severity of the hypertension. Of the studies available, there is a trend towards a worse response to caffeine the more hypertensive you are. Pre-hypertensive individuals show a smaller response to caffeine compared to individuals with severe hypertension when caffeine is consumed. One more factor to consider is the caffeine content in each product consumed. The caffeine content in teas, for instance, is less than the caffeine content in a freshly brewed cup of coffee. Chocolate products are a prime example of variable caffeine content.

In general, there is more caffeine in coffee bean-derived products than cacao bean-derived products. Within cacao products (and there are lots), you have distinctly variable amounts of caffeine and distinctly variable amounts of antioxidants. Hence the effect on blood pressure is expected to vary hugely. So, with the complexity of how caffeine interacts with our cardiovascular tree, how do you know where you stand with caffeine? You would expect the answer to be complicated, wouldn't you? Well, it isn't, really, at least from my point of view anyway. I try to keep things simple, and you can take a dose of my prescription below.

Prescription

I do generally believe people with high blood pressure should avoid caffeinated products with one notable exception: cacao-originated products. I shall discuss the reasons for my opinion on this later.

Now, back to what to do. With so much variability and so many confounding factors in real life, the only way to find out is to test yourself. Yes, it's that simple. Test yourself. When you drink your coffee or caffeinated tea, test yourself by measuring your blood pressure before drinking the beverage as a baseline, then thirty minutes, one hour and two hours after consuming the product. Run the test more than once.

If your blood pressure rises from what it was before consuming the product, then it makes sense to stay away from caffeinated products. Test yourself and find out where you are on the caffeine spectrum.

And test yourself on various products. Do it more than once to exclude a fluke result the first time around. I am suggesting this approach because lots of people are so hung up on caffeinated products, that advice to stay off coffee, for instance, is viewed as heresy.

There are people who believe their life will never be the same without coffee. Would you rather keep consuming a product that sabotages your blood pressure control efforts for the little high you get from its consumption?

Only you can answer that question. Yes, the aroma is awesome. Yes, it does give some level of pleasure. Yes, you get some antioxidant benefits (these are not exclusive to coffee though). Yes, you get a buzz when you drink it. But you can live a reasonable happy life without coffee. It is not the be all and end all. A life without coffee is not necessarily a miserable life. You decide.

CHAPTER 5

What Is Normal Blood Pressure?

Sometimes doctors fail to communicate effectively. "Nothing new there", I hear you say. Communication is an art, and most of us will be continued lifelong learners. That, of course, includes medical doctors too. The way I pass on information to my patients now is not how it was when I qualified thirty-three years ago – a lot has changed. My attention was drawn in my wellness forum to the fact that doctors keep talking about "good control" of blood pressure, yet we do not actually specify what good control is. I suppose, as doctors, we know what we would like a patient's blood pressure to be. But are we telling our *patients* what that is, in a clear and concise manner?

Well, good blood pressure control is getting your blood pressure to what we would consider the zone that reduces your risk of complications from hypertension; the otherwise-known bracket of "normal". Patients need to know and understand that what doctors are attempting to do in terms of good blood pressure control is reduce your risk. That's all.

Because hypertension, just like diabetes, carries risks as baggage. Risks to several organs, in both the medium and the long term. Hypertension will not hesitate to unleash its deadly potential when left unmanaged; it is only a question of time. It patients understood this, and if doctors explained these risks to them, they would be more likely to comply with their management ideas, whatever they may be. This begs the next question: what *is* normal blood pressure?

The world we live in today, at least on the health front, is governed by guidelines. In the US, the Joint National Committee on Prevention, Detection, Evaluation, and Treatment of High Blood Pressure (JNC) under the auspices of the National High Blood Pressure Education Program (NHBPEP) meets every few years to come up with guidelines to assist doctors in caring for people with hypertension.

The NHBPEP's job goes beyond instituting the JNC to reach a consensus on how best to manage hypertension in the ensuing years. The NHBPEP is also supposed to raise awareness in the population of the risks of hypertension, and of the benefits of managing high blood pressure.

The system is no different in the United Kingdom. There is the National Institute for Health and Care Excellence (NICE) which does something similar providing clinical guidelines for medical practitioners in the UK. NICE produces guidelines for management of hypertension to management of diabetes and even guidelines for how women should be looked after in labour.

In the seventh report for hypertension[84], the JNC listed blood pressure readings of between 120–139 systolic (top reading) and 80–89 mmHg diastolic (bottom reading) as pre-hypertension. Readings of between 140–159 top reading and 90–99 bottom reading were defined as stage 1 hypertension. Blood pressure readings of 160 and above systolic and 100 and above diastolic were deemed stage 2 hypertension.

That was then, but recently a new guideline[85] was drawn up jointly by the American College of Cardiology and the American Heart Association. This new guideline re-classified hypertension. In this new classification, normal blood pressure is now considered to be below 120 mmHg systolic and 80 mmHg diastolic, i.e. below 120/80 mmHg. Note the keyword here: "below" – because if your systolic blood pressure reading (top number) is between 120–129 mmHg, but your diastolic reading (bottom number) is less than 80 mmHg, this is considered elevated blood pressure regardless. In other words, a blood pressure reading of 124/72 mmHg is considered elevated. Both the systolic and the diastolic reading must be below 120/80 mmHg to be considered normal.

See the new classification below in one visual guide:

BP Status	Top BP Reading in mmHg	Bottom Reading in mmHg
Normal	< 120	< 80
Elevated	120–129	< 80
Hypertension Stage 1	130–139	80–89
Hypertension Stage 2	≥ 140	≥ 90

What used to be considered as pre-hypertension has now been changed to elevated blood pressure. More importantly, the bar for the diagnosis of hypertension has now been lowered considerably looking at the BP table above. This means a whole lot more people have been dragged into the unenviable world of hypertension using the guide above. And why this change? It is due to an increase in cardiovascular disease complications, as both the systolic (top) and diastolic (bottom) readings get higher. An aggressive approach, therefore, favours mitigation of these complications.

In fact, a 20 mmHg higher systolic blood pressure reading, and a 10 mmHg higher diastolic blood pressure reading were each associated with a doubling of the risk of death from stroke, heart disease, or other vascular disease[85]. Now you can see why it is important to keep a close eye on your blood pressure readings – although not to the point of unhealthy obsession. More about that in a later chapter. Going by the latest guidelines, we should aim to have BP readings of below 120/80 mmHg. That figure will constitute normal blood pressure. But the problem though is asking someone with a BP reading of 180/115 mmHg to get their BP down to below 120/80 mmHg. No mean feat. A lot of folks will struggle to get that low. Making readings of less than 120/80 mmHg a therapeutic target is a lofty idea, but I suspect the reality on the ground is different.

Do not get me wrong. I am all for getting our blood pressures below 120/80 mmHg. But seeing as that goal may be difficult for a lot of people with high blood pressure to achieve, I believe an initial target of 135/85 mmHg is an easier goal to reach. Indeed, in my 2020 wellness forum, I advise individuals to aim for that as a starting point. If most people with moderate to severe hypertension can hit 135/85 mmHg as a first step, then a target that shoots below 120/80 mmHg would not look so distant after all. Little baby steps: a more realistic goal at first, then we can go for that last stretch afterwards. After all, the lower the blood pressure the better.

Speaking of blood pressure readings and normality, you want to ensure that the readings you get are your *actual* readings. This point is very crucial. You will be amazed at how many individuals get it wrong when they are checking their blood pressure at home. Most people have the technique for blood pressure measurement all wrong. What is certainly not pleasing to see is that professionals (some doctors and nurses) get it wrong too. A lot of professionals do not adhere to correct blood pressure measurement techniques, sometimes out of ignorance. Shocking, right?

Let us have a little walk down the blood pressure measuring technique path and you may be able to identify one or two things that you might be doing wrong – as well as one or two things your professional could be doing wrong when he/she checks your blood pressure in the clinic or hospital. Here we go:

Before checking your blood pressure, yourself or with a professional, you must rest for at least five minutes. Rushing into your doctor's office because you were held up by traffic and being directed straight into the office to have your blood pressure checked is plain wrong. That is a recipe for abnormally high readings that do not represent your true blood pressure. You need a pre-blood pressure check rest, either at home when you are doing it yourself or in your doctor's office. This is particularly important.

Next is you sit on a chair that has a back rest. You should place your back on the back rest making sure you are sitting comfortably. Your feet must not be over-hanging. Both feet must be resting on the floor and your legs must be uncrossed. I have a need to always remind myself of this rule, because for some reason I tend to cross my legs once I am seated on a chair. Some habits just creep up on you totally unintentionally.

You want to have your bladder emptied before checking your blood pressure. A full bladder or an urge to want to pass urine even if your bladder is not full will affect your readings. You must not smoke for at least thirty minutes before your blood pressure check. You must not consume any caffeine for at least thirty minutes before your blood pressure assessment. You must not consume any alcohol for at least thirty minutes before your blood pressure check. You must not exercise for at least thirty minutes prior to having your blood pressure measured. Thirty minutes is the official time interval, but personally I believe an hour is more appropriate from my experience.

A good hour is necessary for your cardiovascular system to settle following a workout routine.

When going for your blood pressure measurements at the doctor's office, wear the appropriate clothing. Wear a short-sleeved shirt or dress. The blood pressure cuff should be in direct contact with your bare skin, not over clothing. Long-sleeved clothing is not suitable, as it is wrong to roll up your sleeves when you have a long-sleeved shirt or dress on. A potential tourniquet effect may ensue when you roll up your sleeves, which is a recipe for incorrect readings.

Avoid talking during the five-minute rest interval prior to your check. This should be a complete rest. Crucially, do not talk while your blood pressure is being measured. Professional staff are guilty of flouting this rule a lot – they want to be social, so they initiate small talk during blood pressure measurements. Simply ignore them if they ask you a question, and let it be a one-sided conversation until the blood pressure cuff completely deflates. You can explain to them why you didn't respond when it is over and can apologise if you do not wish to be assumed a rude individual. The arm being used for the blood pressure measurement must be placed on a desk. The arm must be supported with the forearm resting on the table from the elbow.

As you can tell from the above, any professionals checking your blood pressure on the examination couch either in the lying or sitting position with your feet over-hanging and dangling are not meeting the prescribed rules for accurate blood pressure measurement. If your professional is about to check your blood pressure whilst you are sitting on the examination table, you could nudge them in the right direction by simply saying, "don't you think it would be better if we did this on a chair with a back rest and both of my feet on the floor?" If your professional is the humble type, he/she will comply and may even thank you for the reminder. On the other hand, if he/she is the arrogant type, they may continue with the measurement, but you will know better in this instance.

The blood pressure cuff must cover 80% of the arm being measured. The cuff should be placed mid-arm with the lower edge 2–3 cm above the elbow. The cuffed upper arm should be at the level of the heart. Not below it. Not above the heart either. The temperature of the room should be body-friendly: not too cold and not uncomfortably hot either. Noise distractions should be avoided. For instance, loud music. Whether the music is to your taste or not is immaterial; it should be turned off. Any unnecessary background noise must be eliminated or reduced as much as possible.

You will want to take three readings and use the average of the three readings as your index reading for that session. The three readings should be one to two minutes apart. You will notice that the first reading is nearly always the highest. This may be partly due to anxiety; try not to panic when your first reading is high, especially when you are checking your blood pressure at home. See it as something to be expected, as subsequent readings tend to be lower. In fact, I will go as far as saying the first reading should be ignored as it is nearly always anxiety driven. Concentrate on the last two readings as they are more representative. This is my opinion. Not the official advise I should add.

For at home blood pressure monitoring, aneroid and mercuric sphygmomanometers are not ideal. This is because they are clumsy for patients to use alone, and the training required for their correct use is more difficult to master by non-professionals. Therefore, automated devices using oscillometric technology are preferred for home monitoring.

Those are the rules governing accurate blood pressure measurement; you should try to obey all the rules when conducting at-home blood pressure monitoring. I should add that you have a duty to remind professionals of the rules when you observe them being broken as your blood pressure is being measured. The rules apply to everybody: you, your doctor, your nurse. We all want to have correct blood pressure recordings every time, not just sometimes.

The main reason for this is that inaccurate blood pressure data leads to incorrect management decisions. You could be given treatment you do not need if your blood pressure is thought to be high when it is not. In the same vein, you could also be denied the treatment you need because your blood pressure was judged to be low when it was not. Speaking of accurate readings, one often-missed factor is the cuff used for a blood pressure assessment. Cuff size plays a role in what readings you get. There is no doubt that obesity is on the rise, and as we get bigger in size, so do the opportunities to get the blood pressure readings wrong by using the wrong cuff size. Below is a guide on the cuff sizes based on the circumference of your arm.

Arm Circumference	Recommended Cuff Size
22–26 cm	12 x 22 cm (Small adult)
27–34 cm	16 x 30 cm (Adult)
35–44 cm	16 x 36 cm (Large adult)
45–52 cm	16 x 42 cm (Adult thigh)

Here is a question for you if you own a blood pressure monitor. Is your blood pressure machine at home validated? Do not ignore this question because obeying all the blood pressure measuring rules only to use a machine that is not validated is a sin. Yes, it is that serious. This applies to both professionals and home users alike. All machines must be validated to give accurate readings. If a machine is not, then please avoid using it altogether. The need to allow hypertensive patients to monitor their blood pressure at home has created a marketplace opportunity. There is money to be made in manufacturing and selling blood pressure machines, and as millions of people are deemed to have high blood pressure, it is no surprise that many entrepreneurs jumped into the market to get a slice of the cake.

With such an opportunity should come a level of responsibility, or so you would think. Rather, it has opened up an opportunity for some blood pressure machine manufacturers to send into the market inferior products that do not meet expectations. I will try not to paint all manufacturers with the same brush; of course, there are responsible manufacturers who do their best to push quality-assured products into the marketplace.

Anyway, to curtail the chances of inferior blood pressure products stuffing the market, there came a need to have some sort of validation process and procedure. Standards must be set, and standards must be met for all makes and models of blood pressure monitors. That's why, several years ago, the Association of Advancement of Medical Instrumentation, the European Society of Hypertension and the British and Irish Hypertension Society came together to draw up criteria against which blood pressure machines must be measured. It does not matter what corner of the globe you reside in, you should have confidence in the machine you are purchasing, so long as you did your due diligence prior to purchasing. Do not worry – the process is quite easy. A database with all the validated machines is maintained and accessible for everyone to view when needed. This means the list, which is an impartial list by the way, is published on a freely accessible website for the public to view. Each organisation has a website with their own validation list published. All tested blood pressure machines must be entered into the database.

There are protocols to be met in the process of validation. The validation can be done by agencies other than the three official bodies. For instance, the British and Irish Hypertension Society will allow blood pressure devices validated by external agencies to go on its list. But the validation must be independent of the manufacturer. The blood pressure device must pass at least one of the following test standards below to be allowed inclusion onto their database:

1. BHS Protocol (revised 1993)
2. ESH International Protocol 2002 (IP1)
3. EHS International Protocol 2010 (IP2)
4. Universal Standard for the validation of blood pressure measuring (AAMI/ESH/ISO) 2019

The report of the validation test in detail must be submitted to a peer-reviewed journal for publication. The process must be independent of the BP device manufacturer from beginning to end. On the British and Irish Hypertension Society website, they made it possible for website visitors to search by BP device manufacturer, model, type, and validation process. You will also find a list of products that failed the validation test too. Omron is a popular manufacturer, and they do some wonderful products. They have been in the device manufacturing business for a long time. But even Omron does not get it right all the time. You will find some of Omron's products on the list of "not recommended" blood pressure devices. The point being no brand is immune from producing below-par products. This is possibly something to do with quality assurance.

All the resources have similar functionality on their websites. You have no excuse not to check if the machine you currently have at home is a validated machine or not. One also hopes your doctor has a validated electronic blood pressure device too. We frequently advise hypertensive patients to check their machines against their doctor's. It would therefore be a shame if your doctor has a blood pressure machine that failed the validation protocol test.

I have done a video on this topic. If you go on to YouTube and type in the search phrase "is your blood pressure machine at home validated" that video should pop up for you to view the process of checking your machine on those three resources. As said earlier, the three resources below have all blood pressure monitors in databases online. You should easily find out if your machine passed the validation protocol test or not. If your BP monitor is not in any of the three databases or if it is there but failed the test, then you must stop using that machine straightaway. Below are the 3 resources:

http://dableducational.org/sphygmomanometers/
   devices_2_sbpm.html
https://bihsoc.org/bp-monitors/for-home-use/
https://www.stridebp.org/bp-monitors

To round up this chapter, I want to talk about a different way of appreciating what normal blood pressure is. I like to look at blood pressure from the point of view of what the heart is doing. By this I am referring to how much work your heart is undertaking every time it pumps blood out of its bigger chambers (the ventricles). Do not forget that the heart is arguably the most hardworking organ in our body. This is about physical work; hard work, hard labour. Think about it: an organ that is powerful enough to push blood out of its ventricles and force this blood down the arterial tree. That is no mean feat. Not only that but appreciating how often the heart does this is another matter altogether. A cardiac cycle (contraction of the ventricles followed by a relaxation) is a mere 0.8 seconds. That time is made even shorter when there are events demanding that the heart quickens up, like during exercise or when running away from danger. Perhaps we should spare a thought for the heart given the demands on it for our entire lives.

With that picture painted in your mind, you will appreciate what I am about to say next. I like to see blood pressure from the point of view of how much work the heart is doing every time it pumps. Indeed, the blood pressure you get when you check your readings is a measure of how much resistance the heart must work against at that point in time. When your blood pressure is on the normal side, the heart has less work to do. If your blood pressure is high, that means harder work for the heart.

What I have in the image below (Figure 2) tells the story. Please have a good look at the image below first before you continue reading. You need a good grasp of the image to understand what I am going to say for the rest of this chapter. I like graphical illustrations to drive a point home where I can.

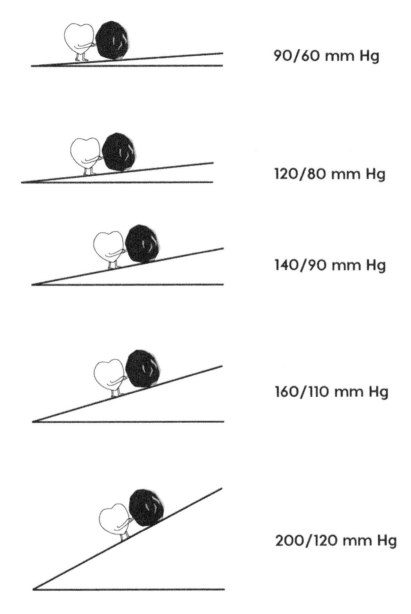

90/60 mm Hg

120/80 mm Hg

140/90 mm Hg

160/110 mm Hg

200/120 mm Hg

Figure 2

Hence, I have come up with a heart and a boulder story line. With every pump, the heart is pushing the boulder. The boulder being the work involved but it is much more than that. The actual work the heart is doing is pushing the boulder up the hill. Pushing the boulder up the hill is representative of how much work the heart is doing, forcing the blood through the arteries against peripheral resistance from these arteries receiving the blood. The lower the blood pressure, the less the resistance from these arteries and consequently the less effort the heart requires to get the blood through.

At low normal blood pressure, like 90/60 mmHg, the heart is doing very tolerable work. Pushing the boulder up the hill easily with little effort. At 120/80 mmHg, the amount of effort the heart needs to push the boulder up the hill is still tolerable. Not a problem at all.

At a blood pressure reading of 140/90 mmHg, that represents the beginning of hard work to get the blood through. The gradient of the hill, as you can see from the image, is just getting a tad steep. There is work required but it is not too sweaty a job. But this is when the heart will start to whine about the job on its hands. The heart does not normally complain unless it sees the need to, and right here is when the moaning begins.

At 160/110 mmHg, the gradient of the hill is now quite steep. The heart has a lot of work to do with this blood pressure. Liken it to pushing the boulder of the hill at 35 degrees Celsius (95 degrees Fahrenheit) heat outside. That is quite some work. It is sweaty work that the heart is doing at this blood pressure, and there is a lot of resistance downstream. The heart is complaining – and justifiably too – that the work is tedious. If you do nothing to flatten the gradient of the hill, and the heart continues to work in these conditions, the muscle of the heart will thicken. Picture that guy who pumps iron in the gym seven days a week, and those bulging muscles he has. That is how your heart muscle will thicken over time. This is what we call ventricular hypertrophy – a thickened and enlarged heart.

Need I comment on blood pressures of 200/120 mmHg? Everything is accelerated at this blood pressure level, and the work is hard. *Really* hard. The hill is very steep, and there is a lot of resistance from the arteries receiving the blood. This is the equivalent of outdoor work, pushing the boulder up the hill at temperatures of 42 degrees Celsius (107 degrees Fahrenheit). The heart has every right to complain non-stop about how much work it is doing at this blood pressure. If blood pressures like these are persistent, heart failure is almost guaranteed over time.

Prescription

If you think of your blood pressure readings in this way, you can see why taking steps to make sure the gradient of the hill is a breeze for your heart would be a reasonable thing to do. Don't worry though, you shall learn about what steps to take to flatten the gradient in the "healing chapters" of this book. Just remember to spare a thought for your dear heart.

Think gradient. Think boulder.

CHAPTER 6

White Coat Hypertension and Masked Hypertension

Given the way world economies are progressing, coins as a form of currency are disappearing fast. There isn't a lot you can do with the lower denominations these days. Thanks to inflation and other economic forces at work. But older folks reading this will know about the concept of a bad penny. For some reason, a bad penny always circulates as currencies do and comes back to you at some point. Central banks do not remove bad coins out of circulation because they are still valid legal tender. That is why the odds are that a bad penny will be back in your hands sometime in the future.

Talking about bad coins, here is a something you should know about high blood pressure. White coat hypertension and masked hypertension are two conditions that make up two sides of the same *bad coin*. They both constitute an enigma. Both masked hypertension and white coat hypertension bring to the fore the imperfections, or should I say *frailty*, of office blood pressure monitoring. Together, they represent a diagnostic and management dilemma that your doctor must somehow confront.

White coat hypertension is when your blood pressure readings are high in the doctor's office, but normal in the community. By normal community blood pressure, I am referring to your blood pressure readings at home. Masked hypertension is the flip side of that bad coin. Your blood pressure is normal in your doctor's office whereas in the community the story is different. Your blood pressure is raised in the community.

What does this mean? It means the diagnosis of the two conditions cannot be dependent on office blood pressure readings. These two conditions represent the need for ambulatory blood pressure machines. Ambulatory blood pressure monitoring is a system of continuous blood pressure checks at pre-set intervals over a 24-hour period using a designated digital portable blood pressure machine strapped on to you. The monitoring could be done for longer than twenty-four hours but currently the 24-hour monitoring is the most common timeframe used by health professionals.

I like ambulatory blood pressure monitoring because it gives a clear picture of how your blood pressure is behaving over a relatively longer period than the usual one-time checks in healthcare offices. When it comes to making decisions regarding blood pressure management, it is imperative that your doctor gets a true picture of your blood pressure over at least a 24-hour cycle. With ambulatory blood pressure monitoring, we can achieve this by continuously monitoring the blood pressure over at least a 24-hour timeline with a view to getting more accurate data.

One of the things I like about ambulatory blood pressure monitoring is that we are offered an opportunity to gather your blood pressure data during your sleep hours. Your blood pressure when you are asleep has clinical significance and I will talk about that in a minute. Another advantage of ambulatory blood pressure monitoring is that we get an opportunity to gather data involving your pulse rate over the twenty-four hours too.

That's not all; data about your blood pressure distribution pattern over a 24-hour timeline can be recorded. The ability to characterise blood pressure circadian variations cannot be overemphasised. The ambulatory blood pressure monitor can be programmed in different ways, the most popular being the ambulatory blood pressure machine is programmed to measure your blood pressure every twenty to thirty minutes during the day and once every hour at night when you are asleep. As stated earlier, the ambulatory blood pressure monitor will also measure your heart rate at the same time as your blood pressure. This gives us a lot of data to work with, meaning doctors can make more effective management decisions.

Wouldn't it be interesting to find out your blood pressure pattern when you are in your office environment? Wouldn't it be interesting to know how your blood pressure behaves when you are shopping in the supermarket especially when you see sudden price changes to your favourite items in the supermarket? Wouldn't it be nice to know how high your blood pressure climbs when you are doing your workouts either in the gym or at home? Wouldn't it be interesting to find out how your blood pressure behaves when you are driving to work especially if your commute lasts longer than thirty minutes?

Wouldn't it be interesting to see your blood pressure pattern when you are doing your daily chores at home? Wouldn't you like to know your blood pressure pattern when you are having your evening meal? Would you like to know your blood pressure pattern when you are watching television or playing a computer game?

These activities may sound mundane or boring, but they do influence the way your blood pressure fluctuates from minute to minute. This is where ambulatory blood pressure monitoring comes into its own; it shows us the correlation between your blood pressure and your daily activities. What's more, we can also get blood pressure correlation with our sleep patterns during non-REM sleep and REM sleep. These are important in managing your blood pressure overall. It helps if, during the 24-hour period, you make notes about what you are doing when the blood pressure cuff inflates. This translates to an easier correlation during the data interpretation process.

Currently, two different diagnostic criteria are available for the definition of white coat hypertension and masked hypertension. It is not noticeably clear which of the two criteria is better, but this is not something you should worry about. This is something your doctor needs to decide, in terms of which of the criteria he/she will apply when he/she receives your ambulatory blood pressure monitoring data.

The first criterion involves using the mean daytime blood pressure readings. This criterion uses the average of the readings from your daytime only. Whereas in the second criterion which has been publicised by the American Heart Association[86] the picture is a lot more segmented. The second criterion involves using three different evaluation intervals.

These are:

1. The mean of the 24-hour blood pressure data in total
2. The mean of the daytime blood pressure values just like in first criterion
3. The mean night-time blood pressure readings

It is not obvious from research activities so far which of these diagnostic criteria has a better predictive value. But the second diagnostic criterion seems to have a lot more going for it. Your doctor will decide which to apply to your circumstances. For instance, it is generally believed that patients with chronic kidney disease complication who have masked hypertension or white coat hypertension will benefit more from using the second newer diagnostic criteria. A recent study[87] showed that mean daytime ambulatory blood pressure monitoring had a better predictive value in chronic kidney disease patients specifically.

Sometime last year I published a video where I talked about the North Star of high blood pressure management. Let me illustrate what I mean by North Star with a little vignette and will explain the link with high blood pressure management afterwards. You know when you go hiking in the woods without the aid of a compass. You are having so much fun in the great outdoors (easy mistake to make) and before you know it, night befalls you. It is foggy. It is windy. The air is muggy too. And now it is dark. It is not surprising that you have become gripped by fear because you are lost in the middle of nowhere without a compass. When fear is in the picture, you could lose perspective especially when you are alone. Thinking becomes a challenging exercise. So, what do you do in that situation where the trees are swinging aggressively with their dynamic shadows gracing your limited view? You must compose yourself, otherwise your cognitive powers will become elusive. You need them. So, hold on to them. You must let go the fear and look for a sense of direction. Remember that you do not have a compass with you, but you need a compass to give you a sense of direction. As it happens, nature does provide us with one: the North Star. The North Star, also known as Polaris, is surprisingly not the brightest star in the sky[88]. It is not even in the top ten brightest stars in the sky, but it has something other stars lack – even the brighter ones. It's a fixed star. The axis of the Earth points almost directly towards it, and as the night progresses, even on such a dreadful night, the North Star does not move.

The North Star does not rise, nor does it set. It is there for you, fixed for you to get your bearings right.

The North Star is a landmark or more appropriately a sky mark. For the 365 days in a year, the North Star (Polaris) is there waiting to guide all of us if we need it. Other stars that may be brighter than the Polaris revolve around it. At any point in the 365 days of the year, the North Star would be visible in the northerly direction. If you were in the South Pole, Polaris would be opposite to your position. Just like it will be directly above you if you stood in the North Pole. The North Star (Polaris) is there to inspire you on a night like this when you feel stranded and all alone. It is your best hope of finding your way home eventually. It is your compass. The North Star gives you a sense of direction. It is your focal point.

So, what has the North Star got to do with high blood pressure? Well, we need to find the North Star of blood pressure management, a focal point. One of the advantages of the 24-hour round-the-clock monitoring of blood pressure is we can see the blood pressure patterns over the entire twenty-four hours. This unique opportunity of ambulatory blood pressure monitoring has given us clues on blood pressure patterns in the population at night through studies.

In truth, most people will have a blood pressure dip at night; this is what research has taught us. This is called night dipping and being a night dipper is a good thing. Being a non-night dipper is, conversely, bad news. This phenomenon of night dipping affects the systolic blood pressure (top number) more than the diastolic blood pressure (bottom number). Most people should see a drop of between 10–20% in their systolic blood pressure readings when they are asleep. These are the night dippers. Others will not see a drop in their systolic readings, and these are the non-dippers. Even worse are the individuals who will see a rise in their systolic blood pressure overnight

– these are the reverse dippers. How do we identify where you belong in these three classes of people? Well, through ambulatory blood pressure monitoring, of course.

Sleep hypertension is common in individuals with sleep disorders, but research has shown that the elderly, those with chronic kidney disease, those with type 2 diabetes and individuals with resistant hypertension have issues with sleep hypertension too[89].

And do you know something else? Mean night-time, asleep blood pressure is a better predictor of cardiovascular disease risk than daytime mean blood pressure readings. Mean asleep blood pressure readings are also an independent predictor of cardiovascular disease risk. A meta-analysis[90] that looked at 302 hypertensive patients with an average age of 69 showed that night-time blood pressure was a better predictor of death and recurrent cardiovascular events in these cohorts of patients. Poorer outcomes were seen significantly more in reverse dippers and non-dippers than dippers, even after adjusting for 24-hour blood pressure.

So, if you are not dipping at night, could you be doing damage to your target organs? One study[91] sought a correlation between non-dipping and target organ damage, looking at the heart as a target organ. The researchers found dippers to have a significantly lower incidence of left ventricular hypertrophy (a thickened wall of the left chamber of the heart). More damage to the heart was seen in those who did not dip at night too. This prompted the researchers to suggest that ambulatory 24-hour monitoring could be employed as a reliable and cost-effective tool to predict and detect early signs of target organ damage.

So, what does this mean? My view is that we should use the management of our night-time blood pressure as our North Star. With so much to focus on in life, zooming in on how our blood pressure behaves at night is paramount. Remember the mean night-time blood pressure remains an independent predictor of cardiovascular risk. Ensuring that your blood pressure dips at night can only be a good thing for your cardiovascular health.

Therefore, controlling our blood pressure at night should be a direct focus for everyone with hypertension. This applies to whatever method of blood pressure control is prevailing for you, be it lifestyle-dominated or medicated. It is the reason I advise taking blood pressure medications at night unless, of course, these are medications that make you pee, or your doctor says otherwise. I know you might be wondering why I am talking about blood pressure medication use when this book is about using lifestyle measures to fix high blood pressure.

I made a video on this topic regarding the best time to take your blood pressure medications. That video has generated some varied comments. Every now and again someone will either leave a comment or email me to ask why I am giving advice on blood pressure medication timing when I should be giving tips on coming off medications. I always tell those folks that I am a medical doctor first and foremost and my duty is to manage risks every day. The last thing I want to do is expose anyone to any unnecessary risk.

Secondly, I live in a world of realism. I know that it takes time for lifestyle measures to kick in. Everyone wants to jump off blood pressure medications as quickly as possible; after two days, perhaps. But, of course, that is not a realistic expectation. Hence, I made the video. Until we get to the promised land, you must use your prescribed medication(s) as instructed.

Prescription

As I stated earlier, if you are not under the constraints of blood pressure medications that make you pee, or are following your doctor's specific instructions, then taking your medications at night or early evenings would be my preferred style. I want us to have better blood pressure control at night. This is the concept of chronotherapy: using the timing of the administration of medications to get better outcomes. For hypertensive individuals, making your night-time blood pressure control the North Star of your blood pressure management is paramount to preventing complications from this silent killer.

Speaking of using lifestyle to control blood pressure, the North Star concept applies here too. I insist we employ methods that target better blood pressure control during the night. My aim is to turn everyone using lifestyle measures to control their blood pressure into a night-time dipper.

CHAPTER 7

Can Lifestyle Measures Fix High Blood Pressure in All Individuals?

I want to talk about the reality of the hypertension world. It is a sizeable part of the planet considering over a billion people have some dalliance with hypertension. This may not be music to the ears of some of you reading this book, but it has got to be said regardless. And it concerns the question: can lifestyle measures be enough to fix your high blood pressure?

Even though everyone with high blood pressure needs help and deservedly so, there are still some obstacles that doctors specialising in lifestyle measures must tackle. And wrestling with resistant hypertension is one such obstacle. What I am about to say next may come across as being negative towards a segment of the hypertension community, but it is the reality as I see it. The segment I am referring to are the individuals with resistant hypertension or what we may describe as "stubborn hypertension". Now let's dive a little deeper into the dynamics of what constitutes resistant hypertension.

Resistant hypertension refers to a situation where an individual is taking three or more blood pressure medications which includes a diuretic (medication that makes you pee more) but your blood pressure is still higher than 130/80 mmHg. We want to help everyone. But unfortunately, not everyone can be helped with lifestyle measures exclusively. The keyword there is "exclusively". Indeed, everyone should use lifestyle measures as a method of controlling their blood pressure regardless of whether they have resistant hypertension or not. We should all be employing these measures to start with across the board anyway. The issue is whether the use of lifestyle measures will be enough to get everyone's blood pressure under control without the need for medications.

As someone who has helped over a thousand people deal with their hypertension issues using lifestyle measures, I have reached the conclusion that people with resistant hypertension will not be able to come off blood pressure medications and rely on lifestyle changes alone to fix their blood pressure problem. The forces opposing your efforts at controlling resistant hypertension with a lifestyle approach are too potent for lifestyle alone to win the battle. The cynic will see this as failure on the part of lifestyle doctors, but it is not a failure, if you ask me; it is more like reality.

Take into consideration the fact that people with resistant hypertension are individuals struggling to get their blood pressure under control, despite being on three or more anti-hypertensive medications. These individuals are taking optimal doses and their blood pressure remains uncontrolled, it is therefore not surprising that lifestyle isn't heralded the hero where conventional medicine has failed. It could happen though, but it would be extremely rare. The best we can expect for individuals with resistant hypertension is a combination of lifestyle applications and blood pressure medications working side by side.

I am a realist. I could sit here and promise individuals with resistant hypertension that their hope lies with lifestyle changes only, but that would be disingenuous on my part and that's not my style.

In dealing with resistant hypertension, our first task is to exclude what we may refer to as "pseudoresistance". Pseudoresistant hypertension is when an individual is wrongly labelled as having resistant hypertension when, in truth, they are not someone who has it. In trying to exclude pseudoresistance, we want to be sure your doctor is getting accurate blood pressure measurements in his office. Is your doctor using a validated blood pressure machine? If your doctor has a validated machine, is he following all the rules for blood pressure measurements? Is he using the correct technique when checking your blood pressure? It is important that your health professional follows the rules of blood pressure measurement, as discussed in the previous chapter.

If you remember, I talked about how getting false blood pressure readings can lead to incorrect management decisions. If your blood pressure is measured *incorrectly* and it is high, despite using three or more medications, then you may be labelled wrongly as having resistant hypertension. This is the reason everybody must use correct blood pressure measuring techniques and that, of course, includes your healthcare professional. If you are indeed someone with true resistant hypertension, the next question we want an answer to is this: are you using your medications correctly, as instructed? The reason this is important is that poor compliance with medication could give the wrong impression of resistant hypertension. Only you can answer that question, and there is a need for honesty here; honesty with yourself and honesty with your health professional.

Ambulatory blood pressure monitoring does help to resolve some of these issues, particularly issues surrounding office blood pressure errors. After all, ambulatory blood pressure monitors will not record false readings over twenty-four hours. With ambulatory monitoring, what you see is what you get. However, if we have confirmed that you truly have resistant hypertension, what can lifestyle measures do to ameliorate the situation?

How about we look out for factors that may be contributing to your hypertension or making the situation worse. If we can hand-pick these contributory factors, then we can target their reversal. No, we will not reverse resistant hypertension by using a lifestyle approach alone, but we can certainly lend a helping hand by fixing certain problems and may be able to meet you halfway with your expectations. One simple objective would be to see if we can reduce the number of medications you are currently taking. Say, for instance, you are on five different medications, we could bring it down to two. I'm sure you would appreciate that.

What kind of contributory factors are we talking about?

Obesity is one to consider. It would be foolhardy to expect conventional medicines to reduce blood pressure in a person whose BMI is 55, for instance. We could try, but I suspect such attempts would be futile. Do you think getting that weight down might offer a helping hand to the medications that individual is using? You bet.

How about someone who doses themselves with lots of processed foods? We all know processed foods come with an enormous amount of salt impregnated into them. Processed foods also have sugar loaded into them and are often infused with fats. When you are flooding your circulation with more salt than your body needs daily, there is a huge sodium load that your kidneys must contend with. This is not fun for your kidneys and is not fun for your blood pressure as a result. I myself do occasionally foray into the world of processed food.

Recently it was my birthday, and because we were in lockdown on account of the pandemic, we got some food from our local Costco store. This included some pizzas. I had not had pizza for a good while, and I have got to tell you that I was amazed by how much salt was in the recipe. It was as if I was shovelling spoonfuls of salt into my mouth with every bite. Taste buds change, and foods you rarely eat will taste different when you eat them several months or years later. It will be a totally new experience altogether, as it was for me on this auspicious day. With every bite, I kept feeling sorry for my poor kidneys, and for my blood pressure hours later. That was a lot of salt. In fact, it was salt overload. Now imagine having to eat foods like that every day, especially when your taste buds have become immune to salt content. Do you really think that being on five or six blood pressure medications will be enough to get your blood pressure down without addressing your salt overload habit? Your guess is as good as mine.

What about alcohol abuse? Someone drinking more than the recommended levels of alcohol daily or several times a week is putting themselves in harm's way regarding blood pressure control. Alcohol abuse is an obstacle that needs tackling to succeed in getting that blood pressure under control. I shall revisit the alcohol topic in the later chapters of this book but for now be aware that alcohol is a double-edged sword with hypertension. Abuse is undesirable. Alcohol abuse will make your blood pressure control resistant to treatment.

Next, we want to address physical inactivity. One of the worst things you can do when you are hypertensive is to be physically inactive. There's nothing hypertension loves more than an affected individual being sedentary. If physical inactivity is left unaddressed, the chances of five medications being successful at controlling hypertension are very slim.

The thing to note here is that individuals with resistant hypertension will have a combination of these factors affecting their lives. It is not inconceivable that an individual weighing 450 lbs could be sedentary, scoffing pizzas every day and have just a little too much love for alcohol. Consider the reality television show *My 600 lb Life*. Consider the lifestyle habits of the individuals you see on that TV show, and you will have a good avatar of what I am talking about.

When issues like the ones above have been addressed, then we can turn our attention to organic causes that may form a valid secondary reason for why hypertension is refractory to treatment. You may remember from earlier chapters that I discussed primary hypertension, or what we call essential hypertension. I also talked about secondary causes of high blood pressure; things like adrenal issues, thyroid problems, kidney problems and even sleep issues, like obstructive sleep apnoea.

Just like we want to address and fix lifestyle-related problems, we equally need to sort out any secondary causes where possible. Failing to do this would mean being in a constant fight with any outstanding secondary causes. In this fight, there is only going to be one winner: hypertension. Is it any surprise that it is resistant?

Here is something I have observed when coaching individuals with hypertension. Those with advanced chronic kidney disease (CKD) are at a huge disadvantage when it comes to fixing high blood pressure with lifestyle measures. My experience is that people diagnosed with chronic kidney disease stages 1 and 2 can have their hypertension reversed; I am a prime example. I belong to the group with chronic kidney disease stage 2. It might take some work, but it is feasible. When you get to chronic kidney disease stage 3, the bar for success is raised further. With CKD stage 3, the best you can hope for is to come off one or two medications. Additionally, there is an argument that individuals with CKD stages 3 and beyond must be on a class of medications thought to protect the kidneys from further deterioration.

These medications are the angiotensin converting enzyme inhibitors called ACE inhibitors and the angiotensin receptor blockers (ARBs). Examples of ACE inhibitors are ramipril, enalapril, captopril etc. Examples of ARBs are valsartan, losartan, telmisartan etc. So, whether we are succeeding or not, being on one medication from one of the two groups of medications is recommended to protect your kidneys if you belong to the chronic kidney disease stage 3 category.

As for chronic kidney disease stages 4 and 5, lifestyle will likely fail as the sole method of controlling hypertension associated with the condition. That does not mean you should ignore lifestyle measures if you have chronic kidney disease stages 4 and 5. You should and must incorporate lifestyle measures but do not expect these measures to successfully wean you off blood pressure medications. In any case, just like in stage 3, you need to be on an either an ACE inhibitor or ARB anyway to ease the amount of protein you lose in your urine and halt further progression of your kidney disease.

Hypertension with associated chronic kidney disease stages 3, 4 and 5 are prime examples of where hypertension is usually resistant to treatment. Doctors often struggle to get a handle on bringing those blood pressure numbers down in people with these conditions. It is nearly always a challenge. Simultaneously though, you also do not want to make things harder for your doctor by remaining overweight, consuming lots of salt, eating lots of processed foods, smoking, drinking lots of sugary beverages and being sedentary. Those lifestyle issues still need to be fixed and doing so will certainly make your doctor's job a little easier.

Prescription

There is usually a reason why high blood pressure is resistant (stubborn) in affected individuals. A search for reasons as to why hypertension is resistant must be made. Sometimes, we may be dealing with secondary hypertension as opposed to primary hypertension (essential hypertension). If your hypertension is secondary, then the issue behind this stubbornness must be addressed if we are to have any chance of success. By that I mean the identified cause must be dealt with and be seen to have resolved before any sustainable consistent blood pressure control can be achieved.

If it is lifestyle-related, then this too needs to be addressed. There is a need to always ask *why* when high blood pressure is stubborn, instead of simply adding more and more medications. Healthcare professionals should always stop and think when faced with resistant hypertension. Simply adding medications repeatedly might seem like a good idea but for every new medication that is added, additional side effects are being introduced simultaneously. It helps a great deal to go back to basics when we are faced with stubborn hypertension.

But I'm also of the view that individuals for whom weaning off blood pressure medications totally is difficult, the least we can do is succeed in reducing the dosages and/or reducing the number of medications they are currently using. That would still count as success, in my opinion.

CHAPTER 8

Your Kidneys – Friend or Foe?

I cannot write a book about high blood pressure and not talk about the kidneys – that would be a sin. And because I intend to go to heaven rather than hell (if you believe in the afterlife), then this chapter is necessary. It can be a little challenging to discuss what I will discuss in this chapter without getting too bogged down in medical terminology, but I shall do my best to keep it light. My objective in this chapter is to help you to understand the kidneys, how they work and how they influence the readings you see on your blood pressure machine.

Enjoy this ride. You are going to love it. Not quite the rollercoaster fun ride you are used to, but you will love it all the same.

The thing is, nature has blessed us with a pair of organs that are vital to life. I suppose you could argue that every organ in the body is vital to life, apart from one little structure. You cannot live without any of your body's organs except one – your appendix. You can live well without your appendix, although you may need it on rare occasions to serve as a conduit pipe in certain surgical procedures. Speaking of vital organs, you cannot survive without your kidneys – period.

As luck would have it, nature has provided us with a pair. It is a good idea to preserve the structure and function of the kidney pair, but you can very well survive with just one kidney, if something unfortunate happened to one of the pair. Located in the posterior compartment of your belly, these two organs do a wonderful job keeping us alive and fresh.

So, what's the purpose of the kidneys anyway? Here are a couple of things your kidneys do for you day in day out:

- Make some specific hormones for you
- Absorb vitamins and minerals for you from their tubular system
- Filter your blood in their rich filtration network system
- Enable you to get rid of waste through your urine

Together the kidneys constitute your body's washing machine. A particularly important job. Because in the absence of that blood sieving and straining functionality, waste products will build up to intolerable levels leading to death. Now you can see why you cannot survive without at least one kidney.

But, of course, the kidneys do a lot more than "wash" and keep our blood clean. The kidneys are also involved in blood pressure regulation – yes, they are. This is where the kidneys can be a friend or a foe, depending on our circumstances.

How Your Kidneys Make Urine for You

In discussing how the kidneys are important to life, we might as well start with their laundry functions. There is a functional unit of the kidney called the nephron. This the little unit that does the wonderful job of filtering your blood. How much blood we carry around in our body depends on our body weight; it is estimated that blood volume is about 10% of your body weight. Every ounce of that blood must be trafficked through the kidneys about twenty-one to twenty-five times a day. That is a lot of blood traffic.

That huge traffic translates to about 180 litres of blood being filtered every single day. And you thought you had a difficult job. Spare a thought for your kidneys, buddy. At least you get paid to do your job. Your kidneys do this for free without complaining too. This huge blood traffic is received by the functional unit – the nephrons. You have about one million of these nephrons in each kidney. How does the blood get to the nephrons? It is through the main artery of the kidney called the renal artery. The renal artery sends out branches which branch out even more getting smaller and smaller progressively until they become uniquely entangled with these nephrons.

These nephrons constitute the filtration system that "washes our blood" for us. Do not be fooled though; these nephrons have much more than filters. They have sensors too. To do its job effectively the nephron has two essential components: the glomerulus and the tubules.

The glomerulus is the strainer, and the tubule is the recipient of this strained blood. The glomerulus strains out the blood into the tubule and in the tubule is where the magic happens. We eat and drink all sorts of food and drink and medications. These are mainly broken down in the liver, and these breakdown products are exported to the kidneys through the blood. The kidney now has the onerous task of cleaning the blood as it passes through the filtration system. It keeps the stuff we need, like minerals and vitamins, and gets rid of the stuff we can do without, like urea (a by-product of protein breakdown) and drug metabolites (breakdown products of medications).

The tubules perform this task of deciding what to keep and what to discard. The wanted are reabsorbed back into the bloodstream for our cells and tissues to utilise. The unwanted products are sent down a kind of sewage system arising from the tubules which ultimately join up to a bigger pipe called the ureter. The ureter is the pipeline that collects urine from the kidneys and sends it down to the bladder for us to void (pee out).

Some of you reading this might object to my description of the kidney to bladder system (the urological tract) as a sewage system. You might see it as overkill when compared to the alimentary system, in which the waste comes out of the back side. Yes, the alimentary system may be a *literal* sewage system, but the urological tract is a sewage system too. It receives what the body does not need in the form of fluid and sends it down the bladder for onward expulsion from the body entirely. Whilst the bottom side gets rid of solid waste from our alimentary system, the bladder side gets rid of liquid waste from the urological system.

This is the reason why it is silly to advise vulnerable individuals to drink their own urine as some sort of therapy for all sorts of ailments. Some will call it traditional medicine, but it is medicine without any common sense behind it. What is discarded in urine is made up of waste products; why on earth would you want to put that back in your body? I have heard of menopausal women who are desperate for relief from their symptoms being advised to drink their early morning urine. It is plain ridiculous, and it will do nothing to help with the menopause.

I suppose the counter argument is that the menopause hormone drug called Premarin is made from horses' urine. Yes, it is true that urine from pregnant horses is collected to make the drug, Premarin. The drug is made by Pfizer. Indeed, the name Premarin is derived from PREgnant MARes urINe. Clever christening, huh? But the urine is refined to extract the oestrogen in it for use in the Premarin's manufacture.

Straight up there, you can see a difference. One urine is from another species that is pregnant, so hormone levels are at their peak, and it is refined to isolate the needed ingredient. The other is from the same species, not pregnant, and unrefined. Being sent straight back from where it came. Besides, as a menopausal woman, your oestrogen levels are low already, hence you have menopausal symptoms. So, you are unlikely peeing out a lot of oestrogens in your urine anyway. Meaning oestrogen concentration in your urine is practically close to zero. Why drink urine that has close to zero oestrogen concentration? Are you beginning to see why that practice is a ridiculous idea? Do not do this if anyone advises you to drink your own urine for any ailment whatsoever.

Alas, I digress. Let us get back on track.

Your Kidneys and Your Calcium Levels

You will recall I mentioned that the kidneys have sensors. One of these sensors detects the levels of calcium in the body. When the kidneys sense that the calcium levels in the blood are low, a chain of events is triggered. One such event is a signal that is also detected by the parathyroid glands. Low levels of calcium trigger the production of a hormone called parathyroid hormone. Parathyroid hormone is produced – unsurprisingly – by the parathyroid glands. The release of parathyroid hormone stimulates an enzyme reaction that causes the kidneys to increase their production of an active form of vitamin D called calcitriol.

When levels of calcitriol are increased in the kidneys by this stimulus, this active form of vitamin D (calcitriol) will stimulate the absorption of calcium from the gut. And that's not all; another action of calcitriol is to prevent the loss of calcium in the urine. This action takes place in the tubules. If you remember, earlier on I talked about how the tubules will selectively choose what to reabsorb back into the blood circulation and what to let go in the urine. The combination of increased absorption of calcium from the intestines and the prevention of calcium loss through the urine means calcium levels are boosted.

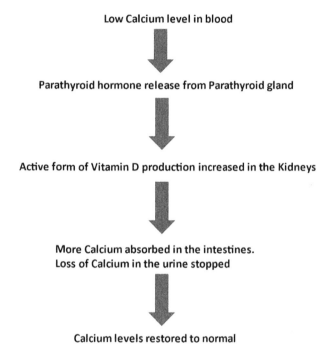

Low Calcium level in blood

Parathyroid hormone release from Parathyroid gland

Active form of Vitamin D production increased in the Kidneys

More Calcium absorbed in the intestines.
Loss of Calcium in the urine stopped

Calcium levels restored to normal

Figure 3

Your Kidneys and Red Blood Cells

Another sensory job the kidneys perform is to boost the production of red blood cells. When the kidneys sense oxygen levels are low, or that the number of red cells is not what it should be, it starts producing a hormone called erythropoietin. This erythropoietin hormone is transported to the bone marrow, where it stimulates the production of red blood cells to restore levels back to normal. Erythropoietin is the hormone that is abused by athletes in their attempts to boost performance. Just a bit of side information there for you.

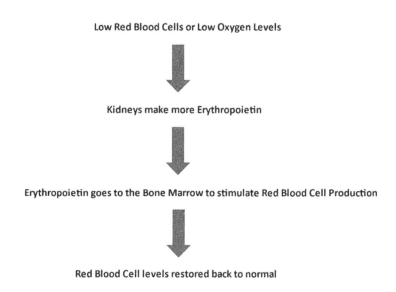

Low Red Blood Cells or Low Oxygen Levels

Kidneys make more Erythropoietin

Erythropoietin goes to the Bone Marrow to stimulate Red Blood Cell Production

Red Blood Cell levels restored back to normal

Figure 4

Your Kidneys, Your Blood Volume, and Your Blood Pressure

The next thing I want to talk about is how the kidneys regulate blood volume and consequently regulate blood pressure on that account. An important function and that is the one that particularly concerns those of us with high blood pressure. There are two ways the kidneys use their sensors to regulate water levels in the blood and our blood pressure. There is the easy pathway and there is the complex pathway. I will start with the easy pathway and save the harder to understand pathway for later. I hopefully will be able to simplify it – fingers crossed.

The Easy Pathway to Make You Pee More or Pee Less

This one involves a hormone called antidiuretic hormone. Let me explain something quickly here. Diuresis means lots of urine production. Diuresis also means you will pee a lot.

Anything that is a diuretic is designed to make you produce more urine and, of course, you are going to pee a lot more. Think alcohol. Conversely, antidiuresis is the exact opposite. Antidiuresis means making less urine meaning you pee less.

So, the antidiuretic hormone does one thing only: it stops you from making lots of urine. How does it do this? Through the kidneys, of course. When the blood vessels – and that includes kidney blood vessels – sense the water level in the blood is low from events such as dehydration and bleeding, or that blood pressure is low, signals are sent to the brain to release the antidiuretic hormone from the pituitary gland.

Once released, the antidiuretic hormone tells the kidneys to reabsorb more water from the tubules – remember those? More water is reabsorbed, and you make less urine. This is the reason your urine gets really concentrated when you are dehydrated. Your kidneys are doing their best to conserve more water to keep your blood volume at its usual levels and maintain your blood pressure at the same time. Blame the antidiuretic hormone.

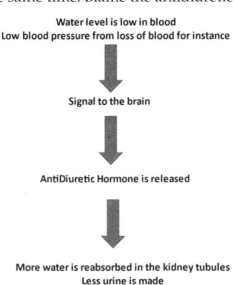

Water level is low in blood
Low blood pressure from loss of blood for instance

Signal to the brain

AntiDiuretic Hormone is released

More water is reabsorbed in the kidney tubules
Less urine is made
Water in blood level restored to normal

Figure 5

The flipside of that coin happens when you have too much water in your blood circulation like when you drink too much fluid too quickly. Signals are sent to the brain to inhibit release of the antidiuretic hormone. Less water is reabsorbed in those tubules. You make more urine. You pee more. Anything that blocks the release of the antidiuretic hormone will make you pee more. Alcohol does a good job of that. So does caffeine.

So, what does water conservation or promotion of water loss mean? It means one thing only: keeping the water levels in the blood the same. That translates into keeping blood pressure where it belongs, i.e. maintaining blood pressure. In this instance, your kidneys are a friend, and an exceptionally good friend at that.

The Complex Pathway That Screws Up Your Blood Pressure

Now, let's turn our attention to the more complex pathway. This is where the kidney is not so much a friend, but more of a foe. It may be for good reason, but it is a devastating turn of events for those of us with high blood pressure regardless. In fact, this second pathway is targeted by a lot of drug manufacturers. Big Pharma tries its best to manipulate this pathway for blood pressure control purposes. There are several blood pressure medications that target different points of this pathway to lower your blood pressure. Whether they are successful at doing this effectively is a story for another day. So, what happens in this complex pathway?

This pathway is called the renin-angiotensin-aldosterone system, aka RAAS. RAAS controls water balance, and also controls blood pressure by initiating the narrowing of blood vessels. The blood vessels that concern us are the arteries; anything that narrows the arteries is bad news for people with high blood pressure. This RAAS pathway is kickstarted by an enzyme called renin. This enzyme was first discovered by two physiology researchers Robert Tigerstedt and Per Bergman from the Karolinska Institute in Stockholm way back in 1898.

Renin is secreted in the kidneys. Renin's behaviour reminds me of a crocodile. Have you ever seen crocodiles in their natural habitat? They give the appearance of being the laziest animal ever created. The crocodile swims quietly in the water. In fact, it glides unnoticed, with no drama when it is swimming leisurely. Even when the crocodile climbs ashore to sunbathe, it gives the impression of being the most laid-back, laziest creature out there. It is harmless in appearance until it is disturbed, or when it goes for prey. That is when you will see the other side of the crocodile; the speed and agility with which it catches its prey or defends itself is something to marvel at. Renin is just like the crocodile: quiet and understated.

Renin release is not triggered until the kidneys sense something is not right. That is when renin springs into action just like the crocodile does when disturbed or going for prey, and this is not good news at all for individuals with high blood pressure. Always remember that the kidney is an exceptionally sensitive organ; too sensitive, if you ask me, but nature knows best. When does renin spring into action then?

1. When the kidneys detect that the salt concentration in the blood is too low. And by salt concentration I am referring to sodium floating around in the blood.
2. When the blood pressure is thought to be on the low side by the pressure receptors in the kidneys based on the amount of blood moving through the nephrons of the kidneys.
3. When there is an increase in sympathetic activity. The worst stimulant is noradrenaline[92].

For those of us with high blood pressure, that third reason is a problem – a serious problem. Do you remember in the caffeine chapter of this book, I talked about how there is always low-level noradrenaline activity going in our body, twenty-four hours a day, seven days a week? You also remember I talked about how people with high blood pressure have a relatively high sympathetic tone. Now you can see why this pathway regardless of whether the first two reasons for renin release are triggered or not, we may still be having some renin activity in the background based on reason number three alone. I do not want to prejudge what happens next, but I have mentioned this earlier on to give you a flavour of how our battle to control our blood pressure is always a true battle as events in this pathway are stacked against us. Anyway, what happens next after renin release is triggered?

Renin acts on a protein produced in the liver called angiotensinogen. Remember that renin is an enzyme, and enzymes are either breaking things down or catalysing a reaction in the body somewhere. In this instance, renin acts on angiotensinogen, breaking it down and converting it to another substance called angiotensin 1.

Ordinarily, angiotensin 1 is relatively harmless to us. That is until it gets converted to another substance called angiotensin 2. The conversion of angiotensin 1 to angiotensin 2 is achieved by another enzyme called an angiotensin converting enzyme (ACE). This ACE is produced in the lungs. Where in the lungs? ACE is produced in the capillaries in the lungs. Capillaries are the tiniest blood vessels in the body. Capillaries have very thin walls. Capillaries are thin for a reason. Capillaries are where oxygen and nutrients diffuse out into the tissues. Capillaries act as a bridge between arteries and veins, so there is a constant stream of blood flowing through capillaries every minute of the day.

When the blood carrying angiotensin 1 passes through the lungs' capillaries, the ACE cells sense it and release the angiotensin converting enzyme. Slight diversion here if I may. The ACE cells in the lungs are attractive to the COVID-19 virus too because the virus latches on to the ACE cells. The SARS-CoV-2 infection process begins once the virus enters inside the ACE cells. But the SARS-CoV-2 attaches itself to another variant of ACE cells called ACE 2 cells. A cascade of events is triggered once the SARS-CoV-2 virus gains access inside the ACE 2 cells. Just a little bit of extra information for you here but let's not get side-tracked as the details of COVID-19 infection do not concern us here.

Back to the RAAS pathway. Once the angiotensin converting enzyme (ACE) is released from the lung capillaries, as blood carrying angiotensin 1 courses through the lung capillaries, it converts angiotensin 1 to angiotensin 2. Remember, ACE is an enzyme. Its job in the instance is to convert angiotensin 1 to angiotensin 2. Are you following the drama so far?

This is where things start to get ugly – really ugly – because angiotensin 2 is one of the most potent vasoconstrictors in the body. A vasoconstrictor narrows the blood vessels: our arteries. Angiotensin 2 production causes our blood pressure to rise, being the vasoconstrictor that it is.

This RAAS pathway is so crucial to how high our blood pressure is regulated from minute to minute and any intervention that breaks it up and stops it from progressing is a fantastic endeavour. Big Pharma knows this. Hence Big Pharma has, and still is, investing millions of dollars into this kind of research. This research targets various points of this RAAS pathway to develop drugs that lower blood pressure by blocking progression of this pathway. Whether Big Pharma has been successful or not is open to debate.

The point of the matter is this: if you can successfully apply the brakes on this pathway at any point, blood pressure will be lowered. Antagonise this RAAS pathway successfully and you are on to a winning formula. Indeed, some of the herbal interventions target the RAAS pathway too just like Big Pharma medications. For instance, if you are using medications like ramipril, captopril, lisinopril or enalapril, the ACE activity in the RAAS pathway is the area those medications are targeting. The idea behind these medications is to inhibit the ACE enzyme from doing its job, hence those medications are called ACE inhibitors. If the conversion from angiotensin 1 to angiotensin 2 does not take place, then blood pressure will not rise. Good so far? Right, let's leave ACE inhibitor medications aside and carry on with our pathway analysis. What is the next task for angiotensin 2?

Not content with raising our blood pressure, angiotensin 2 moves on to the next round and punches us some more. Nothing like kicking a man when he is down, eh? Angiotensin 2 goes to the adrenal glands to stimulate the release of the hormone called aldosterone. Aldosterone, upon its release, springs into action straight away. Aldosterone goes to the kidneys and tells the kidney tubules to reabsorb more water and sodium. The idea is to restore the blood volume to normal, and that action of sodium and water retention singularly causes our blood pressure to rise some more. Never mind the fact that angiotensin 2 is already causing havoc with our arteries by narrowing them.

You now have two synergistic actions in the pathway destined to raise our blood pressure. To complicate things just a little bit more, there is a loss of potassium in the urine too. This lowers the potassium levels in our bodies. You need potassium for good blood pressure control, and we are losing it, courtesy of a conspiracy between angiotensin 2 and aldosterone. It is a battle of wits.

Interestingly, as if the situation is not bad enough as it is, there are other hormones in our body that can activate the

RAAS pathway. Cortisol is one of them, and thyroid hormone is another. Women will be shocked to discover that oestrogen can also activate the RAAS pathway too[93]. Can you block the action of this potent artery constrictor called angiotensin 2? Of course, you can. That is where the blood pressure medications like valsartan, losartan, telmisartan etc. come in. Those medications are supposed to block angiotensin 2 from doing its job. Hence, they are called angiotensin receptor blockers (ARBs).

Another point in the pathway where blood pressure medications can assist is blocking the action of aldosterone. If you are taking spironolactone medication, that is what your Big Pharma is trying to do. I told you it was a complex pathway, didn't I? Hopefully, I have done a good job breaking down a complex RAAS pathway that affects us every minute, every day.

See image below for more clarification:

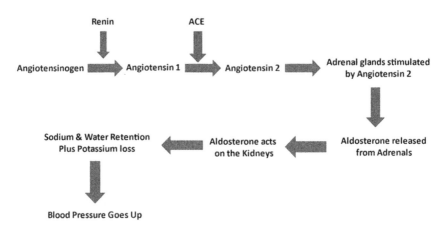

Figure 6

Now you can see what those of us with high blood pressure are up against. This pathway is a pain in the neck. It gets triggered very easily and it is a constant battle trying to quieten it down. In fact, I genuinely believe that individuals struggling to get their blood pressure down to acceptable levels are being sabotaged by this RAAS pathway.

Prescription

We need our kidneys to survive but some of the goings on in the kidneys make our lives difficult. And I am referring to individuals with high blood pressure. It's almost as though the kidneys are conspiring against any move to fight the blood pressure control battle. The renin enzyme, angiotensin 2 molecule and hormone aldosterone are saboteurs in my opinion especially when we already have a high sympathetic tone.

But that's okay. Some of the lifestyle measures I shall discuss in the later part of this book have renin lowering activities. So, do not be disheartened.

CHAPTER 9

Lifestyle Modification for High Blood Pressure – Introduction & Psychology

Let's get down to the real business of managing your blood pressure. Did you notice I said, "managing your blood pressure"? Your blood pressure is like a baby; it needs to be looked after. I will go as far as saying your blood pressure is like a newborn. A baby requires care twenty-four hours a day, seven days a week. A baby is incapable of looking after itself. A newborn needs its parents to care for it, and your blood pressure is the same. Your blood pressure will automatically do its own thing, regardless of whether you ignore it or not. Just like a newborn will cry, pee and poo itself if you ignore it. After all, there is a complex autonomous nervous system wrapped around your blood pressure, influencing how high and how low it goes if you do nothing. You may not like the outcome in this instance though. Your blood pressure needs you 24/7, and it doesn't matter if your blood pressure is in the normal range. You still owe it to yourself to look after it and keep it within that normal range. This is when we talk about a preventative approach.

Of course, the task of looking after your blood pressure becomes a lot more demanding when it is on the high side. You have the bigger job of lowering your blood pressure first and then keeping it in that normal range where it belongs. Successfully lowering your blood pressure is only half the job. Okay, that's a bit unfair – it's three-quarters of the job. You still have a quarter task to execute in maintaining your blood pressure once you have succeeded in lowering it. The reason for this is that if you do not, then it will head up again. I use the newborn analogy because you cannot afford to neglect a newborn, can you? Unless, of course, you are an irresponsible parent.

You may argue that babies do not ask to be born. We bring them into this world, and they are usually planned. You do get the few babies, however, that make their way onto this planet unplanned. Those are the babies that sneak up on you, and they may turn out to be decent human beings who go on to change the world. This is true, and your argument will be that you did not ask for your hypertension; it was imposed upon you. This is true too.

However, now that you have it, you have equally acquired a responsibility that you did not ask for. This is a fact, meaning that looking after it is a task that still needs to be executed regardless. So, let's get over the "why me" whining and just get on with the task at hand. Life is like that: we do not always get what we want, and sometimes we are handed what we do not. So, please do me a favour and think of your blood pressure as a baby that needs looking after. If you think of your blood pressure like that, you will begin to see it in a different light. At least, that's what I did. I had done what any responsible patient would do: looked after my blood pressure as required. I followed instructions. I do not remember my colleagues, who made my diagnosis, telling me anything about lifestyle changes though. That is not so much a criticism than it is an effort to emphasise the zeitgeist at the time. It's now twenty years since I joined the unenviable hypertension club. Has the culture changed? Not much. All I got was a prescription from the onset, which is understandable, considering my race.

People of African descent have been shown to have higher blood pressure readings, and we have an earlier onset of blood pressure problems in life too[94]. Jumping in early with treatment, then, was the right thing to do, but there was a missing link. That missing link is what the rest of this book will be dedicated to. As stated earlier, I followed instructions. I took my blood pressure pills religiously. As a medical doctor myself, I thought it might help if I added some exercises to help with blood pressure control. I knew that, and I felt that I should fall in line, which I did. But there is something called awareness, which you are no doubt familiar with. You would think awareness about an intervention would automatically enable application of that intervention. Maybe but it is not enough in the management of chronic diseases. Being convinced about the effectiveness of what you are aware of is another layer that is often ignored. However, this layer is crucial to the success or failure of that intervention. I call this concept "awareness with conviction".

"Awareness with conviction" is the step after awareness. Awareness simply refers to being in the know about something. Knowing about something does not necessarily equate to knowing how *well* it works. You may have heard that that index thing works but having a conviction about its effectiveness is a totally different mindset. Without moving your awareness to that next step, your belief in the system will be superficial. It will be skin deep, and that is not a recipe for success. "Awareness with conviction" is where it is at. That is where you will find medium to long term results. Anything below that is the equivalent of building a house on quicksand. It is only a question of time before the house comes crashing down.

Here's what I mean. At the time of my diagnosis, I was simply aware exercise was good for blood pressure, for instance. I was aware of that benefit, but I lacked "awareness with conviction" at the time. Based on my superficial awareness, I set out all guns blazing with physical activity. I chose running as my go-to exercise routine and initially it was daily. As luck would have it, I was working in a hospital that was just by the sea front. You couldn't ask for a better location, could you? Jogging by the sea; how cool is that?

My first foray into the world of running was met with some soreness on my foot in the very first week. This was not the usual delayed onset muscle soreness (DOMS); you could expect to have DOMS on the shins, calves or even thighs if you are unlucky, but this was different. It was principally affecting my foot, but I wasn't going to let that get in my way or dampen my spirit. No way. Remember that I was motivated – I was *full* of motivation.

I spoke to a colleague of mine, who suggested I get proper running shoes. She felt the problem was with my shoes. Apparently, you could not just use any pair of trainers or sneakers for jogging. Nope. They had to be shoes tailor-made for running. Don't blame me. I hadn't done any serious exercise in decades at the time, so I simply assumed any nice pair of trainers or sneakers would do. How wrong I was!

Anyway, off I went to the shops. I met a friendly shop assistant, who probably thought *this guy has some money to burn*. She recommended me a pair that would cost me 100 quid. Well, not quite 100, but 99.99 quid – you know the usual pricing gimmicks retailers use. The shop assistant did talk the talk though. I think she sensed that I would purchase anything she recommended – she probably regrets not moving me towards the pairs that cost 150 quid, or should I say 149.99. By the way, we are talking twenty years ago, so a 99.99 quid pair of running shoes was an item some would describe as over the top. I didn't care; I was motivated, and I could afford it. I bought them, and I have to say, they made a huge difference. I felt they were bouncy, although I'm not sure whether that feeling was psychological just because the shop assistant told me they were. Having spent that amount of money, they had to be bouncy. I convinced myself they were. They were certainly more comfortable than my previous pair, and for that amount of money those shoes had to be durable. And you could certainly say they were, but only because they were rarely used after just four months of me buying them.

Yes, four months was how long my romance with running lasted. You know how it goes: you are enthusiastic at first and go out all guns blazing. At first, you're out daily. Then that drops to four times weekly. Then twice weekly. Then once weekly. Then you miss a whole week. You miss two weeks. You miss a whole month and that's it, it's all over. What was wrong there? It's simple. I lacked "awareness with conviction". Instead, I was relying on superficial awareness and motivation.

Motivation is like a muscle. When you use a muscle for exercise, it does get tired, doesn't it? When a muscle is tired, you cannot proceed with the exercise until the muscle has recovered. Motivation is like that. Motivation fills the cup in the beginning and before you know it, the cup is empty. Once the cup is empty, you start looking for excuses not to exercise. And there are a thousand and one excuses out there for you to choose from, ranging from "I have a headache" to "oops, it's raining today, so I won't exercise", even when the weather has nothing to do with your exercise routine. There is something called "home exercises", which the weather outside has no bearing on. Be it rain, snow, blizzard, tornado, or hurricane out there. Okay, that's stretching it a bit – you won't be in the best frame of mind to even do home exercises when there is a hurricane or tornado on the horizon. Your personal safety will be your priority then. But rain or snow? Come on.

Once my romance with the short-lived exercise routine was over, I relied on my Big Pharma medications to see me through. These were medications I took for the next seventeen years until I managed to break free. Coming off medications did not happen overnight. It took some time, but I had to make the decision to take a different route towards managing my blood pressure. I must confess when I took the decision to do something different about my blood pressure, it was a decision I made with a lot of trepidation. And the reason for this is, as you will understand, this approach goes against my training in medical school.

In medical school, we were trained to recognise hypertension as a medical condition that requires treatment with medications for as long as the patient is alive. This meant lifelong treatment with medications, and this was unquestionable. When you have a belief system drilled into the inner recesses of your mind, it is difficult to shake it off. In fact, there were many points in my journey, especially in the first year, where I questioned whether I was doing the right thing. I am sure that if you ask any doctor who has embarked on a similar journey to myself, their experience will probably be the same. It all goes back to our training at medical school. As a doctor, you are taught to diagnose the problem and treat it accordingly with medications. So, when you are confronted with a management technique that is totally different from what you are used to, it takes a lot of mental realignment to accept it. Do not forget that this new management technique constituted a different paradigm altogether for me.

I have been using the word "new" but, in all honesty, managing chronic conditions like high blood pressure with lifestyle changes is not exactly new. There have been pioneers in this field for some time, but I would describe it as new only because the method has not been immensely popular and only a few doctors have used it in the recent past. Yes, it is true that I had seeds of doubt in my mind, especially in the first year of my journey, but somewhere along the line I was convinced I was doing the right thing. In any case, proving to myself that successfully treating high blood pressure with lifestyle measures meant that I could successfully tell people like yourself that the method truly works. After all, what is better than using yourself as a case study?

One reason why doctors – and, of course, that included me – have doubts about the potential of lifestyle changes in managing chronic diseases like hypertension, type 2 diabetes and autoimmune diseases like lupus is because of a lack of awareness with conviction. If doctors are not aware and convinced about the potential of how we can influence disease outcomes with lifestyle changes, then the message will be buried under the weight of our regular medical textbooks. One problem is that having invested so much money in these textbooks and having learnt from them, it becomes difficult to divorce yourself from their teachings. But things are changing, and fast. More and more doctors are getting involved in lifestyle medicine, and that is a good thing. I hear great things all the time from colleagues who are doing wonderful work with patients, and who are getting results even in patients that have been abandoned by orthodox medical practices. There are times when we run out of ideas about what to do next regarding the management of certain conditions in conventional medical practice, and thankfully, sometimes (but not always), lifestyle medicine will come to the rescue where conventional medicine has failed. This is very heart-warming.

We still have a long way to go though. Lots of patients are still uninformed about the value lifestyle medicine can bring to their lives. This is what I would describe as denial of informed consent. One of the things we learnt in medical school is to provide patients with all the information they need. We must tell patients about all the alternatives that are available to them, tell them about the risks and benefits associated with all of the options, and let the patient decide for themselves what is best. One major problem I have identified at the moment is that there is quite a disservice as far as lifestyle medicine is concerned. The message about lifestyle medicine as an alternative is not being provided to patients. You may be surprised to learn that some of the results from lifestyle medicine are comparable to what you see in conventional medicine and – wait for it – without the side effects that Big Pharma pills unleash.

That is not to say Big Pharma medications are not needed. That is not the issue at all, and, of course, there is always a place for Big Pharma pills. However, there is also a place for lifestyle medicine as an option to patients. Wouldn't it make sense for doctors to embrace this and provide patients with the relevant information they need to make an informed decision? Currently, there is a lot of reluctance from my colleagues regarding the success of lifestyle medicine, but how do you know something isn't going to work when you haven't recommended it to patients?

In the case of high blood pressure management, for instance, there is a big space for lifestyle medicine, even in the presence of Big Pharma prescriptions. So, my argument here is that whilst my colleagues are prescribing pills, they should also think about lifestyle prescriptions, or at least consider them. The usual practice of paying lip service to lifestyle prescriptions needs to change. If doctors remembered to include lifestyle prescriptions as part of the package, then lifestyle as a branch of medicine would assume the prominence it deserves.

This is about letting people know what is available, how it is available and where they can access it for their benefit.

I am happy that there are doctors who are setting up medical practices based on providing purely lifestyle prescriptions. In the years to come, as lifestyle medicine becomes more popular and trained medical doctors get involved more and more, we can expect a big change on the horizon. This is my hope, anyway, and I also hope this happens in my lifetime. It is wrong for people to assume, especially when they are young, that genetics have confined them to develop some diseases. This is an extremely popular belief, and my own son believes he is destined to develop hypertension later in life simply because I am hypertensive. This may be true, but it is only true to the extent that he does nothing about it. Live a reckless life, metabolically speaking, and he is destined to get it. The beauty of lifestyle medicine is that it is particularly useful for preventative purposes, just as it is useful for therapeutic purposes.

There is a lot that can be done with nutrition, for instance, but that requires information, and not just any information, but the right information. The internet has made access to information widely available. Unless you live in some primitive society where there is no broadband service, you have no reason not to have information made available to you.

On the other hand, you could be someone who prefers to be denied the beauty of the twenty-first century that is the internet. You know the folks I am talking about: those living off-grid in the middle of the woods. The irony is that those folks tend to be relatively healthy, with the least amount of body fat, and for good reason too. Living off-grid in the middle of the woods is less stressful; those folks are not exposed to processed foods. Instead, they have access to whole foods 365 days of the year. Do I recommend that lifestyle? Maybe, but it's not for everyone. Most of us like our modern conveniences too much to forego them.

The information people need is right at their fingertips via the internet. In fact, these days, the information is available in the palm of their hands. The little device that was originally designed for making phone calls and sending text messages has become a palm laptop. The problem, though, is that it is amazingly easy to get confused with the volume of information out there on the internet. The internet is a wonderful thing, and it has made it possible for information to be democratised, but there is a lot of sifting to do, as information overload is a problem – a serious problem. More importantly, misinformation is an even bigger problem.

Whilst the information is available, and most of it is free, I believe people still need guidance; guidance from the point of view of sifting through the enormous volume and conflicting ideas, and moving away from incorrect information, and guidance from the perspective of applying the right information. Which brings me to the topic of implementation. I can tell you that there are lots of people who believe they are eating healthily based on the information they have obtained free from the internet. But when they learn about the nuances regarding how they can tailor the right nutrition towards what they want to achieve, it is usually an eye opener for them.

Eating right means eating the right foods. Eating right means eating the right foods in the right quantities. Eating right means eating the right variety of foods that supply you with the right nutrients. Nutrients are important; in fact, I would argue that eating foods with the right nutrients is the foundational principle towards achieving good health and preventing and treating chronic diseases. The right nutrients matter more than anything else.

The emphasis should be on getting the right nutrients for the right person. Because if you think about it, how else can you prevent or treat diseases that are amenable to nutritional manipulation without having the right nutrients on board? You cannot escape it; you must have the right nutrients. It is usually an amazing experience when you audit the diet of people who got their information regarding health and nutrition from the internet, only to find out that their nutrition is actually deficient. This is where it is important to have the right guidance, and this requires experience. I am happy to share my wisdom and knowledge with everyone using every medium available. My colleagues pushing the frontiers of lifestyle medicine are also doing their bit to make people aware of what is available to them, and kudos to them too.

Most doctors do not have any significant nutritional training and are therefore not confident in discussing nutrition during consultations. So, expecting good nutritional advice from your physician is expecting too much because you are not going to get it. Your doctor cannot give you what he/she hasn't got. That is not a reason to resign ourselves to doing nothing though. There is something we call multidisciplinary working – a culture that must be extended to lifestyle medicine too. Where we are deficient in a specific skill or training there is usually someone else who has acquired that skill and training. All that needs to happen is for doctors to refer patients to individuals who have the skills and training that they lack. Doctors should not deny patients the opportunity to avail themselves of the services of nutritional professionals, because that is what they are trained for. If doctors feel inadequate from a nutritional standpoint, then it behoves us to send our patients to somebody who can help; a nutritionist or dietitian is just what the patient needs.

As an example, appetite is something that makes people eat and overeat, but it is possible to control appetite when you are exposed to the right quantity and variety of nutrients. The concept of constant dieting and failing repeatedly, therefore, is something that can be solved by simply having the right exposure to the nutrients you need. One of the problems with junk food, for instance, is that the individual overeats because the foods are hyper-palatable. The root of an overeating problem, however, is much more than that. When all you are exposed to is a combination of sugar, flour, salt and oils, your body is going to lack quite a few nutrients.

That nutritional deficiency that results from eating foods containing mainly sugar, flour, salt, and oils only stimulates appetite because your body is essentially asking for the nutrients it needs. Your body is not getting the nutrients it requires, and so will keep craving more food in the hope that the missing nutrients are supplied. Alas, your body still doesn't get the nutrients, and so the craving persists, and the cycle continues. Junk food may be hyper-palatable, but they lack many essential nutrients. That combination of hyper-palatability and nutrient demand is a lethal force on the appetite centres in your brain. Your body will continue to seek those nutrients it lacks until it gets them, hence you feel hungry all the time.

This is aside from the fact that junk food generates free radicals, reactive oxygen species that create oxidative stress and ultimately inflammation in the body. When you eat nutrient-dense foods like kale, broccoli, mushrooms, avocado, celery, watercress, sweet potatoes, mangoes, apples and kiwis for instance, your body will get all the essential nutrients it needs, and that singular action in itself will suppress appetite. This means your body will not crave missing nutrients because it isn't missing any. What's even better is that these foods are energy light, so you don't have to do anything else to manage your weight. Just getting into the habit of eating healthy, nutrient-dense foods is all you need for essential weight management. There is no dieting required and doing this means you can jump out of the yo-yo dieting trap that is all too common.

Your body has an incredible power to heal itself when you feed it well. What we are trying to achieve with lifestyle medicine is to shift the focus of the management of certain chronic conditions away from over-reliance on Big Pharma medications. We are not saying there is no role for Big Pharma medications, however. Of course, there is.

But there is plenty of room for lifestyle modification to play a huge role in how diseases are managed. If you talk to patients who have succeeded in reversing their chronic diseases with lifestyle modification, the joy on their faces is worth a million dollars. The reason for this is that lifestyle modification is, for the most part, free of side effects. The main reason people seek alternative therapy is due to the baggage that comes with using conventional medications, and by this I am referring to the problems associated with side effects. What patients do not like is solving one problem and creating another as a result.

One of the beauties of lifestyle modification is its far-reaching effects on the body. For instance, the effect of eating leafy greens goes beyond blood pressure reduction. These innocent-looking vegetables have effects on the brain, the liver, the kidneys and the heart. When you eat leafy greens, you are doing much more then repairing damage to the walls of your arteries. Leafy greens have phytochemicals that conduct business at a cellular level. They repair damaged DNA, turn off genes that increase your risk of certain diseases and turn on genes that protect us from inflammatory insults.

The beauty of all of this is that these leafy greens are readily available and affordable to most people. Their global geographical spread is quite impressive. However, for people to consume these life-saving leafy greens they need to be aware of their potential benefits. If people are not aware, then of course they will eat minuscule amounts or none at all. When they are aware that these readily available leaves can save their lives though, they are more likely to eat them on a regular basis and in the right quantities.

In the image below I have an illustration of what happens in real life. There is a long queue for Big Pharma and the surgeon's knife. Why is that? Well, these are seen by folks as easier alternatives. Look at the window for lifestyle modification; the staff behind the counter is bored stiff. He has no clients because lifestyle modification requires work – work that people hate. Hence, as humans, we will nearly always opt for the path of least resistance. The path of least resistance is taking blood pressure pills, even if they hate doing so because of the side effects.

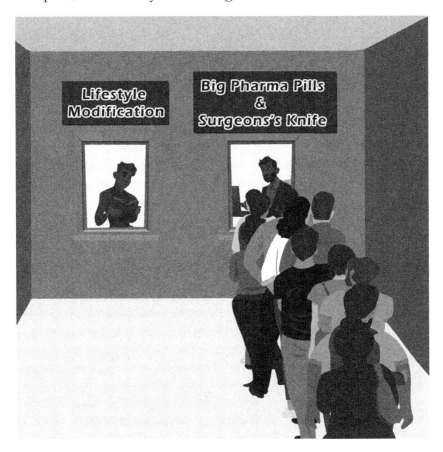

Figure 7

Human beings will opt for pills when given the choice. I opened my wellness forum to the public in the year 2020, with a bias towards managing high blood pressure, although it does cover 360 degrees of wellness in general. This was a deliberate design on my part in order to help people with high blood pressure issues in close quarters. I remember the very first set of questions the first members asked once they had joined. It was – wait for it – "what supplements can I take for my blood pressure problems?" Really? Yes, really.

I was not expecting this. In fact, a video on supplements for hypertension was not one of the videos I uploaded onto the platform while awaiting the arrival of the first set of new members at the time. This is because supplements should not be the first thing to consider when trying to control hypertension with lifestyle measures. However, new members wanted to know this before trying anything else, so I had to quickly put a video together to satisfy their wishes. Human nature, huh? So predictable. The rest of the lifestyle interventions require work, and people don't want to do anything that requires effort; popping pills is easier. And yes, it may be easier, but pills do not get to the root of the problem of hypertension.

Pills, whether in the form of Big Pharma medications or supplements, treat symptoms. The best results are obtained when you combine lifestyle modification with either Big Pharma pills or supplements. What's more, if you are on Big Pharma pills, your next objective is to see how you can have those pills withdrawn from your life for good. There is work involved, I will not lie to you, but if you are prepared to put the effort in, you shall conquer.

What we are good at as human beings is bailing at the slightest difficulty we encounter in any journey we undertake in life. We want it easy. Well, truth be told, using lifestyle modification is simple, but it is not easy. Simple and easy are two different things. Simplicity, in this instance, refers to the ease of the process and structure involved and the ease of understanding it. Easy, however, refers to the simplicity of the process of execution; the process of getting results when you need them.

So, although it is simple to understand the process and get started, arriving at the promised land is not so easy. Results will not come to you while you are lounging on your three-seater sofa doing absolutely nothing; some elbow grease is needed, unfortunately. That is why I say it is simple, but not easy. On the way, there will be obstacles and setbacks. Sadly, most individuals will take flight as soon as they hit the first obstacle; it is human nature to run for the hills and abandon ship when the proverbial hits the fan.

While Thomas Jefferson was burning the midnight oil drafting the Declaration of American Independence, which was later reviewed by John Adams and Benjamin Franklin in 1776, there were diplomatic manoeuvres happening in the background to recognise America as a sovereign state[95]. They did not whimper like frightened dogs at all the hurdles they needed to overcome to realise their dream. If they had, independence would not have occurred when it did. Help from France was particularly important in the fight to gain independence from Great Britain, and it is safe to say that America would not have been an independent country in 1776 had the colonialists buckled at the first bark from Britain. Nothing good comes easy, and you must work at it.

To be successful at using lifestyle measures to control your blood pressure, you must have belief in the system. That's the first thing. I am not suggesting having belief in the system in a "Law of Attraction" kind of way. No, I say this because controlling your blood pressure with lifestyle modifications is a marathon. It is not a sprint event; it is belief in the system that will keep you going. It is what will keep you moving forwards when you do not see your blood pressure dropping to your desired levels after four weeks. If you do not have belief in the system, you will quit after seeing no drop in your blood pressure within an unrealistic time frame. This is what I talked about earlier on; it is awareness with conviction. Having awareness with conviction means you must dream that it is possible. If you do not dream that it is possible, then you are not going to see it through. There is a mental game involved in the process, just like almost anything else in life that requires effort.

This also means you must have a reason for getting into the programme. It could be any reason. It could be that you do not like the side effects of the medications you are currently taking, and that stopping the medications will give you a new lease of life. It could be that you currently feel tired all the time, and that you'll have more energy when you succeed, meaning you can play with your grandchildren on a more practical level. It could be that you just want to protect the health of your brain – don't forget that hypertension has bearing on your brain health as you get older.

How about trying to prevent complications like a heart attack or stroke? How about simply protecting your kidneys from further damage? There are a variety of reasons that should prompt you to want to take control of your health once and for all. It could be a multitude of reasons, or it could simply be one. Either way, you need to have a reason. This is important because without a reason, you may give up when you face obstacles during the journey. I want you to take this point I am making very seriously. You need a "why". You need a purpose. You need a prize. Because when your mind is focused on the prize (or as the saying goes "eyes on the prize") then you are going to have awareness with conviction.

If you do not have a purpose, then your efforts will be aimless. You need a focal point. You need a bullseye. I have taken pains to dwell on this psychological aspect of the management of high blood pressure because I feel it is especially important to get this right from the start. I am hoping that having read this chapter, you will now approach the project with zest and vigour. So, how do you approach replacing your blood pressure medications with lifestyle measures?

Let me lay this out in steps for you:

Step 1

Follow your doctor's instructions and take the medications prescribed for you. Do that religiously and follow any accompanying instructions from your doctor. Be a good patient like I was.

Step 2

Add lifestyle measures. Probably start with about three measures. The reason you start with about three measures is I do not want you to become overwhelmed. We can always add more if things aren't going great.

Step 3

Pump up the volume of whatever measures you have chosen and apply yourself religiously to executing them. No distractions, and always have your "why" in mind. You should have your awareness with conviction by now, and you will know you are doing the right thing. At this point, you should begin to see a positive difference in your blood pressure.

Step 4

Keep a diary of your blood pressure readings. You only need to start doing this when you begin getting consistent normal readings. Keep a record daily for about three weeks. Take your blood pressure readings at the same time every day, preferably in the evenings. If you are not getting consistent normal readings, then you need to add some more measures.

Do not proceed to the next step until you are getting consistent readings that you are happy with. Victory at this stage is especially important, as 60% of hypertensive individuals do not achieve adequate control with blood pressure medications anyway. So, if you are winning at this stage, even if it is with a combination of medications, then know that you are way ahead of 60% of hypertensives who are still struggling despite being on medication.

Step 5

Make an appointment to see your doctor and let him or her know that you have altered your lifestyle and that it is having a positive effect on your blood pressure. As proof of your claim, show your doctor your readings. Request that your medications be reviewed. You do not need to go into details of what you are doing to improve your blood pressure unless you want to. Your results should speak for you.

At this point, your doctor, who is hopefully an understanding individual, will drop one medication off the prescription list (if you are on more than one medication). Or, at the very least, should reduce the doses of one or more medications.

Step 6

Add more lifestyle measures. Add one at a time to prevent overwhelm and keep doing what you were doing before. You should be encouraged by how things are going now anyway. Nothing gives encouragement more than getting results.

Step 7

Repeat steps 4 and 5 once you are getting consistent normal readings again. Over time you will see the next medication(s) taken off the list and eventually you will be medication-free. That is how the process works.

I am of the view that you should involve your doctor in the entire process from the beginning to the end. Every doctor should be happy to see their patient succeed regardless of whatever path the patient chooses. Now let us get into the real business of the lifestyle measures. Below is an overview of the plan for management of high blood pressure. The plan rests on four pillars namely:

1. Diet
2. Exercise
3. Sleep
4. Stress and anxiety management

Everything we do when using lifestyle as a method of managing hypertension rests on these four pillars. If you can win all four battles, your blood pressure is destined to remain low. Of all four pillars, the most difficult is the fourth: stress and anxiety management. The other three pillars can be fixed easily, but stress management remains the trickiest, because life is incredibly stressful on a lot of fronts. Learning to fight stress and keeping it at bay will always be challenging, but it can be done. It may require repeated attempts to deal with it when it rears its ugly head, but I repeat: it can be done.

Prescription

Now I want you to get into the lifestyle modification finisher mindset without complaining. You have high blood pressure. Accept it. A good starting point in lowering your blood pressure with lifestyle measures is to get off the hopeful mindset and get into the finisher mode.

Hopeful mindset renders you powerless. Hopeful mindset makes you unsure. You are without any solid footing. You are simply wishful. You crumble easily in that zone. In that mindset, you are forever wishing and hoping because you are handing over your power to achieve to some other forces. Forces that may never come your way because of over-reliance on expectation than realization. But once you get into the finisher mode, you own those powers and there's no stopping you because you are committed to the cause. Finisher mode means you are taking the bull by the horns. That's the zone for you. Not the hopeful one.

All you need is a plan and I have laid out the overarching steps for you and now you know the four pillars. Yes, the pillars are broad and lack specificity at the moment, so how about we tackle each of them in the following chapters, diving deep into each one. Here's where it gets exciting. Let's go…

CHAPTER 10

Diet for High Blood Pressure

With so many diets available online and offline, this is one area where confusion reigns. When I started my journey, this was the area in which I had the most difficulty trying to make sense of the information I was consuming. Do not forget that even as a medical doctor I had only basic training on nutrition at medical school. That is the way the medical school curriculum is drawn up all over the world; we were taught the basics. This meant that I was starting from scratch in reality.

Like most people with high blood pressure, mine was complicated by prediabetes. This meant that I needed to look for a diet that would help me to prioritise reversing my prediabetes first or, better still, work as a package with my blood pressure reduction efforts. Fortunately, you can kill these two birds with one stone, because for the most part, whatever you do to fix diabetes will also move you along to the hypertension resolution finish line. My diagnosis of prediabetes was the turning point for me to seek a different route for managing my cardiometabolic problems.

At the time, I had hit a crossroads. I was on two blood pressure medications and my own doctor was suggesting that I needed a third medication to have my blood pressure controlled properly. This was a low point for me; my next blood test came back and lo and behold, I had prediabetes. So, we had a situation in which I was on the verge of having a third blood pressure medication prescribed to control my blood pressure and, at the same time, I had developed prediabetes. Nice, isn't it? It doesn't rain, it pours.

It became imperative for me to change course. If I continued on my current pathway of simply taking blood pressure medications and doing nothing else about it, then I was inevitably digging myself into a hole. A big hole, because the likelihood of my also starting medications for blood sugar control in the future was high – very high. This would have made my situation worse, and it was inevitable that I would have developed more complications. In particular, my kidneys were already being blown to pieces by my blood pressure problems. Adding blood sugar issues on top of this would have meant that I was accelerating the process of kidney damage. When you are boxed into a tight corner, you have no choice other than to fight back, which I did.

I decided that I needed to do things differently. Like I said in the preceding chapter, I approached this project with a lot of trepidation. But at this point, I had developed my "awareness with conviction". I had a multitude of reasons. I was focused; I was driven, unlike my first attempt sixteen years earlier when my initial diagnosis was made. You'll remember that at the time, I took up jogging. That attempt lasted just four months. I ran out of motivation, gave up and settled for Big Pharma pills that got me nowhere. This time it was different. There was no stopping me. I had my eyes on the prize.

But on the practical level, I was facing difficulties with my research. There was so much information to consume and a lot of it was conflicting. Conflicting research findings meant I just could not make up my mind what the path going forwards should be. I was desperate to grab the best approach for reversing my prediabetes and in so doing reverse my high blood pressure too.

There is a problem with nutritional research, and you could also say generally in science. There is a lot of corrupt science out there, and this applies to a lot of nutritional research. There are so many vested interests in the subject of nutrition that research findings are usually skewed in favour of the person writing the cheque to fund the research. When commercial interests connive with science, it's a recipe for loss of trust.

If you are someone who has been watching videos on YouTube or doing a bit of research, you will understand what I'm saying. It is not unusual for you to be told that a particular diet is good for a specific medical condition, only to watch another video or read another piece of research that tells you the exact opposite. You don't know who to believe or whom to point the finger at if it doesn't work out as it should. I am not suggesting you turn finger-pointing into a sport, but you get the idea. This was a problem I faced at the beginning, and it took me a long time to decipher the best way to navigate these forests of ideas, permutations, and pathways.

Eventually, I did, but not without making mistakes at the beginning. Don't forget that, at the time, my focus was mainly on trying to reverse my prediabetes. The good news is that a lot of the things you do to manage your blood sugar, whether you have prediabetes or type 2 diabetes, will also positively influence your blood pressure control. As I said, it's all about killing those two birds with one stone. Prediabetes, which is a forerunner to type 2 diabetes, is usually due to insulin resistance. If you fix your insulin resistance, your blood pressure will fall in line. With that in mind, let's see if I can give you some guidance on nutrition regarding controlling high blood pressure.

One question I get asked often is: what is the best diet for controlling blood pressure? For this reason, I am going to discuss some diets. But rather than focus on diets per se, I prefer to talk about the foods that are good for blood pressure control. It will be up to you then to incorporate these foods into any eating plan that you prefer. For me, that is a better approach than trying to fixate on specific, prescriptive diets. However, we live in a world where people are obsessed with this diet and that diet, so I will discuss diets first and then talk about the foods you should be eating. For the most part, the diets people like to talk about with high blood pressure are:

1. DASH diet
2. Plant-based diet
3. Ketogenic diet
4. Paleo diet
5. Carnivore diet

On one count, there were about thirty diets floating around in one form or another, but I will focus on those five above before I talk about the foods you should be eating.

Let's Talk DASH

The acronym DASH stands for Dietary Approaches to Stop Hypertension. This is an eating plan that should be flexible and balanced. The DASH diet is designed to be heart friendly. You do not need to eat any special foods with the DASH diet. The emphasis of the DASH diet is to consume lots of fruits and vegetables. Add whole grains too. You can have nuts, beans, fish, poultry, and dairy. However, the dairy should be low fat or fat-free.

The DASH diet frowns at saturated fat. It isn't saying to avoid saturated fat altogether; you are simply advised to limit your consumption. Vegetable oils are allowed, but tropical oils such as coconut oil, palm oil and palm kernel oil should be limited, because these oils are made up of mainly saturated fats. Fatty meats and full fat dairy are discouraged. Sugar-sweetened beverages, sugar and sweets in general are also best limited on the DASH diet. Reasonable so far? I think it is. A typical weekly serving of foods on the DASH diet is shown below courtesy of National Heart, Lung and Blood Institute resource[96]. This is targeting a 2,000-calorie eating plan per day.

Food Group	Daily Serving
Grains	6–8
Vegetables	4–5
Fruits	4–5
Low fat or fat-free dairy products	2–3
Meat, poultry, fish	6 or less
Fats and oils	2–3
	Weekly Servings
Nuts, seeds, beans, peas	4–5
Sweets	5 or less

The DASH diet emphasises consuming foods high in potassium, calcium, fibre, and protein. Also reducing sodium foods and trans fats foods. The DASH diet has been studied a lot. A study[97] involving 459 adults is one such study. The study participants were fed a typical American diet for a three-week run-in period. They were then randomly assigned to receive the control diet for eight weeks, which was either a typical American diet, a typical American diet but rich in fruits and vegetables, or a "combination" diet rich in fruits, vegetables, and low-fat dairy products with reduced saturated and total fat which is the DASH diet. Salt intake was maintained at constant levels.

The study found that the groups that had the DASH diet as a denominator had significant blood pressure reductions. Just simply adding fruits to the typical American diet was enough to lower blood pressure. However, the group that had the greatest blood pressure reduction was the one assigned to a strict DASH diet. Blood pressure reduction result in the range of systolic dropping by 11.4 mmHg and diastolic blood pressure dropping by 5.5 mmHg in eight weeks is not to be sniffed at.

One of the problems with studies is the lack of good control on the diets of participants. It is difficult to control what people eat when they are in a study when no one is watching. If you did not see me deviate from the study plan, then it didn't happen, right? That is the nature of human beings. You cannot legislate for that. In fact, it is a major confounder when it comes to nutrition research. This does not apply to this study. The foods consumed by participants were supplied by the researchers. That is one major confounder eliminated. Uniformity of foods eaten throughout the study period was guaranteed. I like that about this very study.

What about not supplying the food to study participants and simply give them behavioural advice with or without what to eat with the DASH diet. Offer them advice on other behavioural change like weight loss, increasing physical activity, limiting alcohol intake, and cutting sodium intake. Will that work? This was put to the test[98]. Splitting 801 hypertensive participants with stage 1 hypertension into three groups. One group given behavioural advice only. Second group given behavioural advice but made to implement it and the third group given behavioural advice, made to implement it along with implementing the DASH diet. What the study researchers found was there was blood pressure reduction across all three groups, but the optimal blood pressure reduction was more profound in the group that had the DASH diet included as part of the plan. Over six months of the study, the optimal blood pressure reduction was seen in 35% of the participants in the DASH diet group compared to 19% in the "advice only" group. There are many more studies supporting the effectiveness of the DASH diet. For this reason, when I hear people disparage the DASH diet, I have to wonder what planet they are living on.

There is a medical doctor on YouTube who claims he is yet to see a patient with hypertension improve on the DASH diet. This doctor has an agenda obviously. He wants to be seen as anti-authority. That is how he gets his subscribers. If you position yourself as anti-authority, you can build up a following very quickly as people naturally have a dislike towards authority. It is a perfect marketing strategy. He also has an agenda to promote the ketogenic diet which he prefers, and benefits from, but that is the world we live in.

Now Let's Talk Ketogenic

We might as well talk about the ketogenic diet seeing as it is the favourite diet for some of my colleagues. I say, some, not most. If there is any diet that has caused so much controversy on this planet, the ketogenic diet will take some beating. The controversy surrounding the ketogenic diet has been ongoing for years, and it isn't going anywhere soon. This is mainly because there are ongoing concerns regarding its effects on health, in particular on blood lipids. It is a concern that is difficult to ignore, I must confess, and is one reason why I departed that camp. But that's just me: a cautious doctor. You may be one of those who is in love with it, and good for you. Good luck to you in the long term too.

The ketogenic diet, as it was originally conceived, was a diet that was low in carbohydrates, had an adequate proportion of protein and had a high fat content[99]. The diet was designed to treat stubborn epilepsy in children with recurrent seizures that were unresponsive to conventional medicine. And it worked; the children placed on the ketogenic diet had fewer and fewer seizures whilst on the diet, and this seizure-control effect lasted even after the diet was discontinued[100]. In the absence of an adequate amount of glucose, which is the body's preferred substrate for energy needs, the liver has no alternative than to turn to the substitute nutrient available to meet demands for energy. That substitute nutrient available is fat, and the supplies are in abundance with the ketogenic diet. The liver converts the fats from the diet to fatty acids and ketones.

The body's tissues will consequently use the ketones for energy supplies. A multimillion-dollar industry has sprung up from the popularity of the ketogenic diet, a growth that has been helped immensely by social media. Some companies have even made it possible for you to just drink commercially available ketones. Spare your liver the ordeal of converting consumed fat into ketones; why bother? Give your liver a break and let it rest. Why not just drink ready-made ketones and run your body on them? I am not kidding – there are plenty of ketone supplements about. Now you see why the ketogenic industry will do everything in its power to defend the ketogenic diet as the "best diet" for any medical condition under the sun, including asthma. Yes, asthma. Go figure!

As you can guess though, surviving on a carbohydrate content of 20 g or less a day is a challenging enterprise. That's because most of the foods that are readily available to us today are carbohydrate-based. This diet requires discipline – a lot of discipline. Although, by definition, the carbohydrate quantities per day can go as high as 50 g, as per the original concept of the ketogenic diet dreamt up in the early part of the twentieth century. In practice, however, the typical ketogenic diet of the twenty-first century targets 20 g per day. This is because the typical ketogenic diet is really a "very low carb, high fat" diet. One apple is all you need to hit the suggested ceiling of 20 g per day. Consume more than an apple and you're already crossing the line towards getting kicked out of ketosis. Of course, there are variations of the diet, and one that readily comes to mind is the Atkins diet. I am not a fan – or should I say I am no longer a fan – of the ketogenic diet. It was the first diet I tried out when I started my journey, and the idea of avoiding carbohydrate foods, given my prediabetes predicament, was incredibly attractive at the time. As expected, I was angry with carbohydrates for "giving" me prediabetes, so it made sense to kick them out for good. It was nice to eat foods that didn't have blood sugar spikes as a background concern. I ate lots of fats and lots of protein too. This was what I thought: throw carbs away and everything will be just fine. Except it wasn't.

I struggled to get myself into ketosis for weeks, despite my best efforts. I was sabotaging myself with the amount of protein I was consuming. Protein will get converted to sugar eventually, and you will be kicked out of ketosis if you were already there running on ketones. Either that or you won't get into ketosis at all. There is a lesson there for those of you who may be fans of this diet. If you are struggling to get yourself into ketosis, you may want to re-evaluate your protein intake.

I was frustrated, but over time I got the hang of it and finally hit ketosis. Staying in ketosis, though, was another battle. I suspect I was not consuming enough fats, because deep in the inner recesses of my mind I had a fat hesitancy too. The gospel was to eat plenty of fats. This is true. But you need to be careful when you are doing a ketogenic diet and you already have cardiovascular issues. I could not overcome my fear of turning my blood lipids into weapons against my fight to control my blood pressure. The ketogenic diet would have enabled me to peg my blood sugar and have a brilliant HbA1C – but at what cost?

A hike in my LDL-cholesterol? This was not something I liked. More importantly though, the ketogenic diet makes insulin resistance worse. Yes, you may get good blood sugar readings and a nice HbA1C to show for it, but it's just a façade. The ketogenic diet does not address the root cause of your pre-diabetes or type 2 diabetes. The root cause is insulin resistance, and the ketogenic diet papers over that problem. It's a band aid, a plaster on a wound. Why do I say this? It's quite simple, and to prove it, here is a little test for you. If you are on a ketogenic diet, have a ripe banana and see how your blood sugar responds. Your blood sugar will hit the roof. That's because your insulin resistance is worse than it was when you started, and the ketogenic diet makes you more carbohydrate intolerant. When I was on the ketogenic diet, I dared not have a ripe banana, but now I can eat four bananas in one sitting and my blood sugar will be fine. Why is that? It's because I have addressed my insulin resistance problem and have made myself more insulin sensitive. I didn't achieve this on the ketogenic diet.

As you will have gathered, my ketogenic diet experience was not a pleasant one. I needed to change course… again. And I did. But you don't have to; if you are comfortable with your ketogenic commitment, unlike me, just be aware that the ketogenic diet does not address the root cause of your blood sugar issues – insulin resistance. You will remain extremely carbohydrate intolerant if all you do is run your body's systems on ketones ad libitum. Does the ketogenic diet help with weight loss? Absolutely, if it's executed correctly. I say this because for all its successes in helping people to lose weight, there are countless numbers of individuals who struggle and fail on the ketogenic diet too. You could argue that this applies to all diets, and that is true too. I will concede that. This systematic review[101] of thirteen studies comparing the ketogenic diet with a low-fat diet gave the ketogenic diet a thumbs-up over the low-fat diet. The reviewers also showed that the ketogenic diet reduced diastolic blood pressure. What explains why ketogenic diets induce weight loss? There are a couple of explanations.

One is that the protein content of the diet causes satiety[102]. I am sure you have noticed this yourself, regardless of whether you are on the ketogenic diet or not. When you consume a meal with relatively high, decent protein content, you feel fuller for longer. A protein meal within a range of 25–81% has been observed to cause enough satiety, even with a single meal, to lead to an overall reduction of energy consumption[103]. There is also the thinking that ketogenic diets suppress ghrelin, the hunger hormone, when users are ketotic[104]. One study comparing a ketogenic diet with a medium-carbohydrate, high-protein diet suggested suppression of appetite and lower energy intake in the ketogenic group as a mechanism of action. The principal mode of action being a direct appetite suppression by the ketone bodies produced as a result of using fat for fuel[105].

Another study which was more or less a carnivore diet with no carbohydrate at all (30%, 0%, and 70% of energy from protein, carbohydrate, and fat, respectively) in comparison with a normal diet composition (12%, 55%, and 33% of energy from protein, carbohydrate, and fat, respectively) confirmed production of new glucose in the body (gluconeogenesis) when the body is deprived of carbohydrates[106]. Reduction in the production of new fat cells and breakdown of existing fat was the explanation in that study as the mechanism for fat loss and this review agrees too[107].

Another review[108] offers a different explanation as to why weight loss occurs with a ketogenic diet. It suggests the production of new glucose in the body from sources other than carbohydrate as a catalyst for fat loss. The theory being that producing new glucose (gluconeogenesis) is a metabolically expensive project that uses up a lot of energy. It also says the metabolism of proteins themselves uses up a lot of energy, hence inducing an energy deficit, and consequently fat loss.

Does Your Body Still Need Glucose at All When on a Ketogenic Diet?

Talking about gluconeogenesis, why does the body need to bother about making new glucose when it is already running on fats? This is all about homeostasis. Although your body is burning ketones for its energy supplies on the ketogenic diet, this does not mean it will allow your blood glucose levels to plummet to zero. Your body will still need to maintain some glucose levels in the blood, even if it is at the most basic level. You will always need a baseline glucose amount in the blood, twenty-four hours a day, seven days a week. That's just the way it is; run on ketones all you like, but regardless, you still need to maintain some glucose balance. For that reason, your body will generate glucose from either protein or fat stores, or the fat you consume in your ketogenic diet. This is irrespective of the fact that you are not using this glucose primarily for your energy needs. You could say the body needs a backup system in place just in case you falter in your supplies of ketones. The longer you have been on the ketogenic diet, the less glucose you generate as you become keto-adapted.

Keto-adaptation refers to when your body has completely adapted to burning ketone bodies for fuel and you become less reliant on glucose. Once you fail to supply the required amount of fats to make enough ketones though, or once you consume too much protein, the glucose generation machine will be fired up and you will be kicked out of ketosis. That's why people who love their bacon and steak too much whilst on the ketogenic diet find themselves being kicked out of ketosis more often than they would like. The keto-adaptation interval can take anywhere from four to twelve weeks. It took me six weeks when I did it.

Prepare to have the keto flu whilst keto-adaptation is going on. Keto flu is not nice; you will most likely experience issues like nausea, difficulty sleeping, headaches, brain fog, irritability, fatigue, and constipation, usually within two days of starting the ketogenic diet. This keto flu may last up to nine days, and sometimes it is bad enough for people to quit the process altogether. You can accelerate the keto-adaptation period, though, by including intermittent fasting in your ketogenic enterprise.

The fact that the ketogenic diet precipitates weight loss is not disputable. Most people agree that weight loss occurs with the ketogenic diet, and sometimes rapidly too. This would explain why the ketogenic diet might be adopted as an option for blood pressure control. Any intervention that facilitates weight loss will result in a blood pressure reduction. How much reduction will vary from one person to the next.

The next viable question though, is this: do these folks on a ketogenic diet keep the weight off after the initial success? For most dieters, the challenge is not losing weight in the short term. In fact, practically all diets make weight loss possible in the short term. After all, why call it a diet if it doesn't procure any fat loss upon its execution. The real challenge is what happens in the long term. We do not quite know what successful weight loss maintenance means objectively. We know what it means literally but what about objective definition? This paper[109] proposed a definition of 10% weight loss and keeping the 10% off within a time frame of twelve months as a minimum. That bar is quite low in my books but even if we run with this as a standard, a lot of keto dieters still fail the test.

The reason for this failure is that the ketogenic diet is quite restrictive. Most people will fail the long-term test easily; with so many carbs around, the power of carb seduction after seven months of carb deprivation, for instance, is usually too much for people to resist. It is not surprising then, that many keto dieters fall by the wayside after a couple of months. They are deemed to have failed the yo-yo test. The penny seems to have dropped, and keto dieters are realising how difficult it is to remain compliant in the medium to long term. Yes, there are some hard-core ketogenic dieters who go all in, if you like, but the vast majority usually succumb to the lure of carbs eventually.

Ever Heard of Carb Cycling?

So, what can we do? Enter the concept of carb cycling. The original idea behind carb cycling was to optimise energy on workout days, having carbs on workout days and switching back to a ketogenic way of eating on other days. A carb cycler flips between a high fat and a high carb diet. In my view, carb cycling is an admission that carbs are essential to life, and it is always a bad idea to cut out an entire food group for whatever reason. I am not a fan of cutting out an entire food group – that's not my style!

There are different formats to carb cycling. Some people will do one week on keto and flip back to high carb the following week. Some will do one month of keto and another month of high carb eating. Or two months keto and one month high carb. I have seen different permutations of this diet-straddling formula and there is nothing wrong with that. Dieters should be free to manipulate a diet to suit them.

Does changing a strict ketogenic diet to a carb cycling formula affect weight loss efforts though? A group of researchers have tested this out. They placed overweight participants on a staged diet protocol over a period of twelve months using the Mediterranean diet as the index diet. The cycling format the researchers opted for was twenty days of ketogenic Mediterranean, twenty days low-carb non-ketogenic, four months Mediterranean normo-caloric nutrition, a second twenty-day ketogenic phase and then six months of Mediterranean normo-caloric nutrition[110].

It definitely looks complicated, I know, but the cycling protocol worked. The study participants dropped an average of 16 kg in weight with an average drop in percentage body fat of 10%. Even secondary parameters like LDL-cholesterol, triglycerides and glucose levels improved over the twelve-month period. This research tells us that ketogenic dieters do not necessarily have to run their bodies using fat as their single energy source. Opening themselves up to the option of re-introducing carbs like sweet potatoes, oatmeal, beans, peas, lentils, wholegrains and even fruits intermittently does work, and doesn't detract from the anticipated benefits of a ketogenic diet.

One advantage of carb cycling is that it obviates one of the major headaches of weight loss, something we refer to as metabolic adaptation. Metabolic adaptation is probably best known in popular terminology as starvation mode. Metabolic adaptation occurs when your weight plateaus because your basal metabolic rate shrinks following a rapid weight loss. Your body is trying to hold on to the fat it has left and is saving it for a rainy day (these days never come in modern life). It is all about saving the fat for that anticipated period of calorie restriction that occurs during starvation, rather than burning it. When this happens, your weight loss flatlines, which can be very dispiriting and frustrating.

In real terms, for example, let's imagine you are on an 1800-calorie diet and are doing fine. Your weight is coming off gradually and you are feeling good about your progress. Then, all of a sudden, your weight flatlines on the 1800-calorie diet. To see any more progress, you will need to drop your daily caloric intake some more, probably to 1600. That human protective mechanism is what we call metabolic adaptation, and it affects most people on any weight loss journey. Your body is holding onto what it has got once it senses what you are up to. Our bodies are really smart at detecting accelerated weight loss.

Metabolic adaptation also affects your energy output too. Meaning an exercise regime that was working for you earlier in your journey also stops paying off. You will need to increase your exercise output to kickstart your progress again. It is thought that when you carb cycle, you calorie cycle too by default. So, on your high carb days, you should be consuming more calories than your high fat low carb days. Dialling your calories up and down means your body will fail to recognise that you are trying to lose weight. Therefore, will fail to switch on the metabolic adaptation button. Lucky you!

The second advantage of carb cycling is it is also thought to prevent leptin disruption. Leptin is a super hormone that has influences on other body hormones and our metabolism as a result. Leptin is produced in fat stores, and it is an outreach hormone that influences how our brain views our metabolic status[111].

The more body fat you have the more leptin you have. A high leptin level tells your brain to stop making hunger hormones that will make you eat more simply because you have enough stores for that rainy day. Conversely, when you drop your fat stores through dieting, your leptin levels drop too. The idea being to inform your brain to push an agenda for hunger to make you eat more and replenish fat stores. What this research[112] is also telling us is that dropping your carbohydrate intake fuels a fall in leptin levels. The idea again is for the body to protect the body's carbohydrate stores by encouraging you to eat more, preferably more carbs.

With carb cycling, you prevent that fall in leptin induced by an exceptionally low carb intake on the ketogenic diet. By raising your carb intake through carb cycling, you reset your leptin levels. You stop hunger pangs as well as pause a further fall in leptin. Every time you introduce high carbs, you press the leptin reset button and your leptin levels increase.

There is research evidence to support the practical point that carbohydrate overfeeding (high carb eating), but not fat overfeeding (high fat eating) is what increases leptin levels[113]. It therefore makes sense to embrace carb cycling if you want to adopt or are already using the ketogenic diet as a means of weight management to help your blood pressure reduction efforts.

Now Let Us Talk Paleo

The full name for the Paleo diet is the Palaeolithic diet. Another name for it is the ancestral diet. As the name implies, this is a diet that is taking us back to our distant past. It's a nostalgia diet that transports us back to what we ate when civilisation was nowhere in the horizon.

The Paleo enthusiasts believe in making us take a practical historical journey back to when we ate what we hunted. The hunter-gatherer ideology. The belief is that we ate a lot more healthily then in contrast to today's foods that are heavily processed and making us sick. The background ideology from the Paleo camp is that if we go back to 10,000 years ago and ate like our ancestors at the time, we won't have all the modern-day diseases that are plaguing us today. Hence the synonym for the Paleo diet being the Ancestral diet.

If you think about what the Paleo folks are saying, they do have a point. They are right from the point of view of our ultramodern diet making us ill. That's true but in making that comparison, they are making a serious assumption too. The Paleo folks are making an incredible assumption on the health and well-being of our ancestors. Were our ancestors always healthy? The evidence from mummies examined from different regions of the world does not appear to support that claim. There is this interesting study[114] where whole body CT scans were performed on mummies from four different geographical regions of the world. Making sure mummies in the study were from both sides of the Atlantic. You will be surprised to learn that there was evidence of atherosclerosis (hardened arteries) in mummies from all four regions; and that included the pre-agricultural hunter-gatherers too. This finding casts serious doubt on the claim that diseases like atherosclerosis that cause heart disease and strokes are modern diseases that were completely absent during pre-historic times.

Paleo folks believe that the Neolithic period which followed the Palaeolithic era ruined our health by providing humans with foods we were not designed to eat. One good thing about humans is that nature gave us a brain that does more than let us plan our next hunt. No one can argue that our evolution over the years has helped to advance humanity. Think about modern technology and how we enjoy these conveniences today. Of course, in tune with human advancement, we felt that hunting every day was not a practical way to source our food. We needed something more reliable, something that would provide us with a constant and uninhibited supply of food 365 days a year. Enter modern farming. Sadly, this is what the Paleo brigade have a problem with. Paleo folks believe that modern agriculture is the foundation of most chronic diseases; at least the common ones, anyway. Therefore, a retreat to the Palaeolithic era's way of eating is their proposed solution to our diet-induced diseases.

Paleo followers hate beans. They hate peas. They hate lentils. They don't like starchy root harvests like potatoes, and they avoid dairy like a plague. They hate grains, and naturally they have a problem with grain-derived foods such as cereals. I will agree with them on the dairy and cereal front, but don't touch my legumes, potatoes, and grains. Those I have to disagree with. The Paleo diet focuses on meats, fish, fruits, nuts, seeds, eggs, and vegetables. These are officially allowed foods. A recurrent problem with diets like Paleo as you can see from above is that they are unduly restrictive. With restriction comes difficulty with compliance in the medium to long term.

Some modification of the diet will go a long way to improving long-term compliance. In my opinion, there is nothing wrong with adding legumes to the Paleo diet. It not only gives the user a bigger span of foods to eat, but a more inclusive diet that provides more nutrients. The Paleo diet lacks adequate fibre and adding legumes would go a long way towards boosting this dietary deficiency. I do not want to go into the benefits of fibre here but suffice it to say that fibre is essential to good health.

Does the Paleo diet reduce blood pressure? A small randomised three-month crossover study comparing response to Paleo diet and the standard diabetic diet based on dietary guidelines showed promise[115]. There was a small reduction in diastolic blood pressure as well as improvement in blood sugar parameters compared to the standard diabetic diet. There are lots of studies supporting the effectiveness of the Paleo diet for improvement of type 2 diabetes. With type 2 diabetes being a sister problem of high blood pressure, it will be reasonable that blood pressure improvements are a goal within reach on Paleo.

What About the Carnivore Diet?

If you thought the Paleo and ketogenic diets were restrictive, think again. There is always an outlier that goes one better.

Enter the carnivore diet. This one is super-restrictive – if you stick to the original concept, that is. The carnivore diet has its legion of super fans and celebrity promoters. Two that spring to mind are a popular orthopedic surgeon and a popular psychologist. These two folks have been on YouTube and the radio and have featured on blogs and podcasts extolling the virtues of the carnivore diet. Convincing? Yes, they are. If you are reading this book and have spent any reasonable length of time online, you probably know the individuals I am talking about. I do not want to mention their names as they may not approve of such publicity in a book. So nameless they shall be, but you know who.

The psychologist talks about how his daughter, who had a terrible time with an autoimmune disease, tried everything else and nothing appeared to work. It made her deeply unhappy. Then she tried the carnivore diet and has never been happier or healthier. In fact, the story is that she introduced her father, the psychologist, to the diet by telling him about her results. He got into the diet and his life was transformed as well. He succeeded in finding a resolution for his depressive symptoms with the carnivore diet, according to him. What about the orthopedic surgeon? Well, he heralds the carnivore diet as a life saver too. There is a video of him on YouTube talking about how he is the only 50-something year old who can dead-lift a certain amount of weight. I can't remember the precise figure he quoted. He does look well-ripped and muscular. He may also have abs that you could ride a bike on without breaking them, but there are a lot of 50-something year old individuals with a similar physique who can dead-lift enormous weights too.

There are similar transformative stories dotted about the internet about the successes of the carnivore diet. On that basis, it is difficult to ignore such testimonials. People do lose weight on the carnivore diet, there is no doubt about that, but it is not always plain sailing. There are failures too – just as there are with all diets. One reason for this is the restriction, which makes compliance a mountain to climb. The carnivore diet is arguably the most restrictive diet out there.

Speaking of restriction, what can you eat on the carnivore diet? Before I talk about the foods allowed on the diet, let me clue you in on one big selling point of the carnivore diet, or any restrictive diet for that matter. The carnivore diet makes shopping for food easy. You don't have a lot to think about when making your food purchases. The problem with a multiplicity of food choices is one less thing to worry about with the carnivore diet, because you need only concentrate on meat and organ meats, and you are done. Seriously, what could be easier than going to the supermarket and picking up duck, chicken, beef, lamb, eggs, goose, pork, ox, fish, shellfish, goat, turkey, liver, kidneys, heart, lungs, lard and tallow? That's essentially all you need to put in your shopping cart; maybe add some seasoning and you're off. It couldn't be easier. Choose whatever meat or organ meats you're craving that day, pick up some seasoning agents to make the meat palatable and your shopping is done.

I do remember the psychologist saying in one YouTube video that all he eats is beef, salt (salted beef that is) and water. That's it. If all you ate were different meats or organs with different seasonings to add variety to the taste, I would imagine that the idea of fat loss would not be far-fetched. If you can put up with the boredom of just eating that way for the rest of your life, then your fat loss issues are resolved forever. And if the weight falls off, usually your blood pressure will follow, within reason. So, there is an argument that the carnivore diet is one route to reversing high blood pressure. Just remember though, the benefits of the carnivore diet have more to do with what the user is *not* eating than what they *are* eating. A restrictive diet, like the carnivore way of life, is certain to induce calorie deficit just by the sheer nature of its structure.

Being so restrictive means processed foods are off the menu. What is the commonest cause of metabolic dysfunction leading to chronic diseases like type 2 diabetes and hypertension? Processed foods. Eliminate processed foods and you are straightaway on to a winning streak regardless of what name you slap on the diet. An off-shoot problem with restriction, just as in the Paleo situation, is the potential to run into difficulties with nutritional deficiencies. I did talk about fiber issues in Paleo. The same applies here. Vitamin deficiency may be an issue here with the carnivore diet. The kidney as organ meat does not have vitamin C as far as I know but apparently the liver has vitamin C and B6. Who would have thought? But could you eat liver every day for your vitamin C daily needs? Regardless of getting a couple of vitamins from the liver, a carnivore dieter will be missing out on phytonutrients which are solely available from plants only. If you think that's an accept-able price to pay, then stick with it.

If you are going to embrace the carnivore diet, a reasonable thing to do would be to let your health practitioner know about your new style of eating. Some level of health monitoring will be essential to ensure you are not lacking in some vitamins or minerals. More importantly that health parameters like your blood lipids are not spinning out of control. I believe that an extra level of protection is necessary given the limited nature of the carnivore diet.

Never Forget Plant-Based Eating

Unless you have been living under a rock or locked yourself in some far away forest log cabin (and who can blame you for doing such a thing in our modern-day crazy world) you would have heard the phrase "plant-based eating" in the last two decades or so.

Yes, plant-based eating is alive and well and it's almost seen as the boxer in the blue corner of the boxing ring whilst the ketogenic diet represents the boxer in the red corner. The debate has always been between these two diets. And you could lose your mind if you try to keep up with the mudslinging that goes on between the proponents of both diets fighting it out in every public forum known to twenty-first century planet Earth inhab-itants. It's a never-ending fight with each diet being self-righ-teous. Both deeply entrenched in their positions. None of them prone to any movement of any sort to meet each other halfway.

You could argue that these deeply entrenched positions may be related to commercial interests on the part of some individ-uals in this never-ending debate, and this occurs more on one side of the fence than the other. There are a lot of commercial interests to protect on the ketogenic side of the argument, and when you have science to support your arguments, it becomes apparent why you may not want to move your position. There's always science on your side if you look deeply enough though; whether that science is bias-free is another matter.

Cynics will say that when you have always held a belief, and if your livelihood also rests squarely on this belief, then changing your position may amount to "betrayal" of the cause and a destruction of your bottom line. You will stand firm, even in the face of newer scientific evidence that tells you your position is wrong. Such is the situation in today's world. Call it cognitive bias or call it cognitive dissonance. It's your choice. Let's cast the mudslinging and mentally exhausting exercise of who is right or wrong in the ketogenic/plant-based diet debate aside and dive a little deeper into plant-based eating styles. After all, we have already talked about ketogenic diets, and it would be unfair not to discuss plant-based eating, as I believe it is very relevant to blood pressure control.

Truth be told, every diet is blessed with merits whilst carrying its own weighted cons. Some have a disproportionately heavier weight of cons than others, in terms of health outcomes. There is no such thing as a perfect diet, at least not in the way popular diets have been designed, anyway.

So, What Is Plant-Based Eating?

If you went to a shopping center and randomly asked a hundred people what plant-based eating is, I would hazard a guess that ninety-five of those individuals would tell you that it is veganism. Why is that? It's because people equate plant-based eating with veganism, but the truth is that the two terms are not necessarily synonymous.

Vegans represent one end of the spectrum of plant-based eating, but they do not represent all plant-based eating. Plant-based eating is a much broader term; all vegans are plant-based eaters, but not all plant-based eaters are vegans if that makes sense. On the spectrum of plant-based eating, you have people who get 85–95% of their nutrition from plants and the rest from animal products. These folks tend to keep animal products within touching distance, and this varies between individuals in the framework.

For instance, we have the vegetarians who will eat dairy from animals and exclude all other animal products. These are the lacto-vegetarians. There are folks who will have eggs but no dairy – the ovo-vegetarians. There are the ones who will have both dairy and eggs and no other animal products – the lacto-ovo vegetarians. You also have people who believe anything from the sea or of aquatic origin is fair game, such as fish and seafood but won't eat poultry or red meat. They represent the pesco-vegetarians by classification. Finally, you have folks who will eat all of the afore-mentioned foods, spiced with a dose of poultry. However, they keep poultry to a bare minimum, such as once or twice a month. These folks consider themselves plant-based eaters too, although any vegans reading this will be screaming "murderer" at this concept.

The point of the matter, really, is that plant-based eating is a diverse way of life in which the bulk – and I mean the *bulk* – of the foods you consume consists of plants. Plenty of plants. The diversity of this way of eating comes from the potential to add varying types and amounts of animal products. In truth, a low frequency of animal product inclusion is to be expected in plant-based eating. You may have plants only, the 100% fully plant-based eater. And you could also have a variation where animal products constitute a very small percentage of your nourishment. That's the beauty of the diversity of plant-based eating. It's a broad church with plants constituting the foundation and structural bricks and mortar, if you like.

I do not think we should be judgmental about where on the spectrum of plant-based eating someone stands. Some people do very well on a 100% plant-based diet, but there are also individuals who simply fail to achieve the lofty heights of feeling good and looking well eating just plants only. These are the folks who, for one reason or another, feel that the introduction of animal products in small doses helps them to achieve better well-being.

We are all different, and sometimes our genetics make it impossible for us to feel well eating 100% plants only. Have you ever met a pale and weak-looking vegan? I have met one or two. These individuals find it difficult to exercise routinely as they are always tired. On the other hand, we have vegans who really thrive on the diet, and some are body builders with crisp, well-chiseled bodies. You could say the vegan diet was designed for these folks. It is also possible that the weak vegan may be eating predominantly wrong vegan foods. It is always assumed that all vegan way of eating is healthy. Not really. Brownies, cookies, biscuits, crackers, cakes, sodas, and fruit juices are all vegan foods. Are these healthy foods? No, they are not the last time I checked. If you decide to go vegan and concentrate on these highly processed vegan foods, you will be courting health problems. Without doing a thorough food audit, it is difficult to ascertain why an individual may be failing to bloom and flourish on plant-based eating.

So, what constitutes a healthy plant-based eating? Plant-based eating that will pass rigorous scrutiny should have plenty of whole grains, legumes, vegetables, and fruits, as well as nuts and seeds. All of these will be included, with or without small amounts of animal products. The distribution of these foods will vary between individuals and will vary on different days in one's diet. A prerequisite for success in plant-based eating is for an individual to have a variety of these foods daily. A decent plant-based eating plan should have a good spread of different foods to avoid nutritional deficiencies, especially in those who are strictly vegan.

This might be an appropriate time to talk about the nutritional deficiencies that may occur with the vegan lifestyle. These deficiencies will probably be less likely if animal products were included in the diet. I suppose the counter argument would be, if a vegan did that, then that diet wouldn't be vegan any longer, would it? So, maybe that wouldn't work here because the strict vegan diet is more than a diet. It is a lifestyle that goes beyond food. It is a belief system that thinks of animal welfare in its entirety. A vegan will not attend an entertainment show that involves animals, for instance. Think circuses and rodeos. A vegan wouldn't wear clothing made from animal fur. Veganism is a lifestyle. It's beyond diet!

As a prelude to what the next few paragraphs entail, I should re-emphasise that a good spread of plant variety in plant-based eating is particularly important to prevent nutritional deficiencies.

Now, let's talk about possible nutritional deficiencies that could occur with the type of plant-based eating that cuts off food groups and how to deal with them. Remember I said plant-based eating is a spectrum of eating. Veganism is one end of the plant-based eating spectrum. Veganism, in the strictest form, can potentially lead to one or two nutritional deficiencies, hence worth discussing here to alert those who may wish to become vegans for control of blood pressure purposes. I am paying particular attention to plant-based eating because this is the diet that has been shown through several studies to reduce the risk of cardiovascular events.

This is the diet that I recommend for anyone who wishes to control their blood pressure naturally. Whether you include a small proportion of animal products like eggs, yogurt, fish, and seafood will be up to you.

Plant-based eating is particularly good for blood pressure control, and I would encourage you to adopt it as someone reading this book. But at the same time, I do not want you to fall into the trap of nutritional deficiencies that could occur. Adopting a style of eating that is beneficial for your blood pressure should not come at a price.

Personally, I do not think adding a small amount of animal products to your plant-based eating plan would detract from the results; so long as you are adding whole foods. Adding Greek yogurt, for instance, will not affect your blood pressure reduction efforts. After all, the healthy yogurts, like Greek yogurt and plain natural yogurt, are fermented, and fermented foods are good probiotics which are beneficial to gut bacteria which in turn benefits us. It is unlikely a plant-based eater will have issues with calcium deficiency if a small amount of dairy in the form of natural or Greek yogurt is added to the overall eating plan. I am not suggesting you eat that every day, but it helps. Calcium deficiency is seen often in strict vegans, but lacto-vegetarians don't seem to have that issue.

I should mention that the calcium deficiency in vegans has a lot to do with not having a good spread of plant foods in their diet. But at the same time, dairy is a reliable source of calcium in the diet. If excluded completely, then there is a chance of calcium deficiency. You need about 1000 mg of calcium per day in your diet. If you avoid dairy altogether, then you need to include the leafy greens like kale, watercress, turnip, and collards in your plant-based eating quite often to get adequate calcium.

If you are not keen on a small amount of dairy, you could also get some calcium from plant-based milk like almond milk, cashew milk, hazel milk but you should ensure it is a calcium-fortified milk. How about ensuring you get foods like okra, beans, almonds, edamame and, of course, soy products. Including these foods in your eating plan and cooking your leafy greens which promotes absorption of the calcium will ensure you avoid calcium deficiency.

Vitamin B12 is another nutrient that may be lacking in 100% plant-based eating. The reason for this is that plant sources of vitamin B12 are woefully unreliable. There is some suggestion that algae such as spirulina and chlorella may have vitamin B12, but this is conjectural and is likely not reliable enough to be a recommendation for plant-based eaters. The vitamin B12 found in spirulina was initially thought to be the real B12, but the latest evidence seems to suggest that it is instead a pseudo-vitamin B12[116]; this means it is a vitamin B12 analogue, and it is not bioavailable to humans[117]. Wherever you have biological analogues, expect competition for the receptor sites of the biological molecules. It is therefore now thought that the potential competition for receptor sites between the real vitamin B12 and the pseudovitamin B12 in spirulina could have the potential to cause vitamin B12 deficiency. Could you take vitamin B12 supplements to avoid this risk if you are using spirulina? Maybe. Until we have some solid research backing for this, my view is to avoid using spirulina, and if you do use it, do so sparingly. And as for chlorella as a source of vitamin B12, the jury is still out on this at the time of writing.

The generic advice currently is that those who are strictly vegan should use vitamin B12 supplements. This advice is even more relevant if you are taking medications like proton pump inhibitors which block acid production in the stomach. Proton pump inhibitors are medications like omeprazole, lansoprazole etc. Any medication that blocks acid production in the stomach will require you to check your vitamin B12 levels often; especially in older folks whose acid production is not that efficient any longer compared to their younger days. Acid in the stomach is essential for vitamin B12 (cobalamin) release from vitamin B12-containing foods. This is the first step in the vitamin B12 absorption process. So, anything that inhibits acid production in the stomach also reduces vitamin B12 absorption by extension. If you are using these acid blocking medications, I suggest you get yourself vitamin B12 supplements. It's important you do.

Another nutrient deficiency that a strict plant-based eater may encounter is omega 3 fatty acids[118]. They are a very important and essential group of fatty acids. We need omega 3 fatty acids for all sorts of bodily functions; not least being the foundational ingredient of some of our hormones' production and being an integral part of the structure of the cell membrane. Omega 3 fatty acids also play a role in how our cell receptors behave. Omega 3 fatty acids exhibit anti-inflammatory effects. Omega 3 fatty acids perform important functions in early life – docosahexaenoic acid (DHA) plays a role in the visual and neurological development of the foetus and the growing child. Quite apart from slowing down our cognitive decline, omega 3 fatty acids may assist type 2 diabetics improve their blood triglyceride levels. There are some suggestions that omega 3 fatty acids may play a role in the relaxation of our arteries too, therefore, potentially helpful in lowering blood pressure.

What is clear is that omega 3 fatty acids are essential fatty acids, meaning our bodies cannot synthesise these fatty acids. Any biological molecule that our bodies cannot synthesise has to be either obtained from food or from supplements. We can do just that by getting omega 3 fatty acids from either our diet or from supplements. Therein lies a potential problem for plant-based eaters who are strict vegans, if they are not taking omega 3 supplements. Let me explain.

There are three omega 3 fatty acids:

1. Alpha-linolenic acid (ALA)
2. Eicosapentaenoic acid (EPA)
3. Docosahexaenoic acid (DHA)

DHA and EPA are obtainable from fish sources. Usually oily fish like mackerel, herring, salmon, oysters, anchovies, sardines etc. hence both DHA and EPA are called marine omega 3s. ALA is available from plant sources like walnuts, flax seeds, flax seed oil, other nuts, chia seeds etc. The problem though is the body does not use ALA directly. ALA needs to be converted to either DHA or EPA for our body to utilise it properly. EPA and DHA are longer chain omega 3 fatty acids, and our body seems to prefer the longer chain omega 3 fatty acids to meet its needs. Sadly, the conversion output is poor. Below 5% conversion is suggested by studies[119]. Only a small percentage of ALA is converted to EPA which is unfortunate. Worse still is that conversion of ALA to DHA is worse than conversion to EPA although gender differences exist[120]. Men have a rougher ride with the conversion. Women win the battle of conversion here probably because of the influential oestrogen hormone[121]. What happens to the rest of the ALA we eat then, if only a small percentage of it is converted into EPA and DHA? Well, you'll be glad to know that the unconverted ALA isn't wasted; it is processed into energy instead.

Do omega 3 fatty acids have an influence on blood pressure reduction? There is evidence that they do. We know from earlier that DHA and EPA are the two fatty acids the body prefers to utilise, right? Well, this meta-analysis[122] pooled a number of randomised controlled trial studies together and examined the effect of EPA and DHA without upper dose limits – and including food sources – on blood pressure.

The study found a very modest reduction of blood pressure in people who did not have high blood pressure. Even better news is that EPA and DHA did reduce blood pressure a little bit more in people who had high blood pressure and weren't on treatment. A 4.5 mmHg drop in systolic blood pressure reading (upper value) and an average of 3 mmHg reduction in the bottom value (diastolic). Remember these were untreated individuals. I should point out that doses of more than 2 gm are required to see reductions of diastolic blood pressure. A similar study[123] looked at using 1 gm/day of EPA and DHA for cardio-protection and higher doses for blood pressure reduction.

The point here for the strict vegan is that the ALA you consume may not be enough to supply adequate amounts of EPA and DHA which our body prefers to use because of the poor conversion rate. This translates to potential omega 3 deficiency even though you may be consuming enough ALA from your diet. You could, of course, get your EPA and DHA from supplements, or you could be flexible in your dietary approach as a plant-based eater by including oily fish in your portfolio in order to get those two fatty acids directly from their natural sources. Just a thought.

Do plant-based diets provide blood pressure reduction benefits? Of course, they do and there is plenty of evidence to support this. If I may quickly draw your attention to another study[124], which gave participants a prescribed plant-based diet that consisted of raw fruits, vegetables, seeds, and avocados for just over a four-week period. The researchers obtained anthropometric and hemodynamic data weekly, inclusive of baseline data over the four-week period. The researchers found outstanding blood pressure reductions. Would you be happy with a 16 mmHg reduction in your systolic readings and a 9 mmHg reduction in your diastolic readings just from eating plants? I am sure you would, and not only that: you have the potential to reduce your blood pressure medication burden, just from eating mainly plants!

Prescription

Your primary objective in your choice of diet is to pick one that will move the needle on the weighing scale. Shedding just 10 lbs of fat will have a significant positive impact on your blood pressure. More importantly, your diet choice should help you maintain your weight once you hit your target and should not have any negative impact on your blood lipids.

An equally relevant point to consider is blood pressure control is a long-term commitment. It is not a sprint and that should influence your choice of diet. Is it a diet you see yourself doing in five years' time, ten years' time? This is not a quick fix before heading back to square one as is always the case with most people. We are not interested in short-term gains and long-term losses here. This is a lifestyle change. In fact, I will suggest not subscribing to "a diet" but rather a way of eating – a way of life instead.

My prescribed "diet" is a plant-based way of eating or the DASH diet as they meet those objectives very well but feel free to make any choice that suits you better but remember the aforementioned caveats.

CHAPTER 11

What To Eat To Fix Your High Blood Pressure

From the preceding chapter, we already know that eating plants is the way forward. Regardless of the diet you choose, making plants the bulk of what you eat is the way to go if you want to naturally lower your blood pressure. I can attest to that, and you will find out for yourself in the course of your blood pressure lowering journey. If you think about it, most Big Pharma medications are synthesised from plants, or from what you may otherwise call botanical sources. These may be land or marine plants, and usually, the pharmaceutical industry identifies a specific phytochemical in a plant, zooms in on it, extracts it, refines it and voilà, you have a medicine.

Of course, I have oversimplified the process here, as there is a lot of testing and trialling involved. The later aspect of drug trials is focused on efficacy and safety, and lots of data need to be collected on both counts. Regulatory bodies will need this information before a drug is finally approved. If we know that plants have nutrients and phytochemicals inside them that are good enough for drug research and development, why don't we just go directly to the source and eat the whole plant? Are you now beginning to see where I am coming from? Controlling your blood pressure will require eating a variety of plants in your overall diet plan, and the more plants you have in your diet, the more widely you are casting the net in order to capture active ingredients with pharmacological activity. Hence, overly restrictive diets miss out on low-hanging fruit opportunities (no pun intended) for blood pressure control. Think about it: what one plant lacks, another will probably have in abundance. A good spread of plant foods is therefore paramount.

Eat plants, folks. Eat plants!

Yes, we will add some animal products so that we balance our nutrition, but the focus should be principally on plants. So, the next question is, what plants should you eat to get your blood pressure under control?

Answer: eat plants that are rich in:

1. Antioxidants
2. Potassium
3. Nitrates
4. Magnesium

There are other nutrients that may add some leverage to what we want to achieve but focusing on those four nutrients will go a long way to getting us to the promised land. If we want to split hairs, I will add that antioxidants are a group of phytonutrients as opposed to just one single nutrient. Now, let's talk antioxidants…

Foods Rich in Antioxidants

If there is any reason why we should preserve biodiversity everywhere on the planet, it is that plants are the hub of anti-oxidants and therefore need all the protection they deserve.

There are other reasons, of course; not least the importance of biodiversity in protecting the environment and halting any further deterioration of our climate. Plants remain our main source of antioxidants, and they are a cheap source at that.

Plants naturally possess antioxidants due to the stresses of their environment. It is their way of protecting themselves from the nasty realities of harsh environmental conditions. Their adaptive response to the environment is our gain. We can access these exogenous antioxidants from plants such as spices, mushrooms, traditional medicinal plants, fruits, vegetables and even flowers.

So, what are these natural antioxidants? Examples of these will be:

- Phenolic acids
- Flavonoids
- Anthocyanins
- Carotenoids (carotenes and xanthophylls)
- Lignans
- Stilbenes
- Glutathione
- Coenzyme Q10
- Lipoic acid
- Phytoestrogen
- Catechins
- Vitamin C
- Vitamin E

The above is not an exhaustive list; there are many more natural antioxidants. Lots more. What do these antioxidants do? To talk about the uses of antioxidants for us as humans, we must go back to why they are important and why they are needed in the first place. Just as plants are subject to environmental stress, so are we. Think cigarette smoking, air pollution from car emissions in congested cities, industrial emissions from our hyper-productive world, radiation, alcohol. Even the UV rays from the sun constitute an environmental stress for us. And that's not all. The minute-by-minute metabolic processes going on in your body as we speak generate stress too. Plus – wait for it – exercise is also a stressful factor. Can you believe that? Yes, it's true, but it's a welcome controlled stress.

What do these stressful events produce? They generate free radicals in the body, sometimes called reactive oxygen species (ROS) or reactive nitrogen species (RNS), such as superoxide and hydroxyl. These free radicals are electron "thieves"; they are oxidisers, they search for electron donors (reducers) in the body. Unfortunately, many of our bodies' tissues and biological molecules are happy to donate electrons to these eager thieves. When you have an eager thief and a donor willing to leave the door open, it's a marriage made in heaven. This simple act of generosity is bad for our health. For instance, if LDL cholesterol donates electrons to these electron thieves, it becomes oxidised. Oxidised LDL cholesterol is the cholesterol that embeds itself in the walls of our arteries. This oxidised cholesterol is an active participant in the cascade of inflammatory events that lead to plaque formation: the process that causes damage to our arteries.

These free radicals (ROS and RNS) can also alter the way messages in the DNA of our cells are transcribed. Bad transcription messes up the DNA, and these free radicals can also alter what goes onto the surface of the cell and the membrane surrounding the cell. The implication being that what the cell sends out and what the cell takes in is altered by these free radicals. As you can see, free radicals have the potential to cause chaos in the way our body functions. Free radicals are the vehicles for the chronic inflammation implicated in chronic and degenerative diseases including cancer. In our case, the chronic inflammation that destroys our arteries also leads to the hardening of our arteries, and the net result is high blood pressure. What the antioxidants do is donate free electrons to these electron-hungry free radicals – also called oxidants. This prevents our cells and circulating biological molecules from becoming donors and, in doing so, protect our health. Normally, the body can dispose of these free radicals with ease; nature has systems in place to create a fine balance between oxidants and antioxidants. But exposure to environmental stresses tilts the balance in the direction of excess oxidants, and this is the origin of a lot of our metabolic diseases; excess oxidants floating around our bodies is a nightmare. We therefore need a buffer for these oxidants: we need electron donors, and plenty of them. Having these exogenous electron donors (antioxidants from plants) will optimise our health and reduce our blood pressure.

So, if we increase our consumption of antioxidants through proper nutrition, we arm ourselves with these able reducers (electron donors). We halt the initiation, multiplication, and proliferation of oxidative chain reaction. These antioxidants will help us to mop up the free radicals, thereby putting out the fires caused by oxidative stress. Reduced oxidative stress is good for our arteries and, therefore, good for our blood pressure. Now that we've cleared up the pro-oxidant and antioxidant systems and how both systems operate, let's turn our attention to what foods we should be eating to obtain these generous electron donors.

Foods rich in antioxidants include:

- Brussel sprouts
- Broccoli
- Blueberries
- Red cabbage

- Spinach
- Artichokes
- Sweet potatoes
- Squash
- Collard greens
- Pumpkins
- Beets
- Beans (all types)
- Kale
- Raspberries
- Goji berries
- Strawberries
- Pecans
- Dark chocolate (90% or higher)
- Red grapes
- Carrots

That's a good list for you. Get started with those and see how your blood vessels will become more pliable and elastic.

Foods High in Potassium

There are four nutrients that were recently identified to be lacking in the diet of Americans. Potassium was one of them, as found by the Dietary Guidelines for Americans 2010 Advisory Committee[125]. Only a mere 3% of Americans met the recommended intake of potassium in the 2003–2006 NHANES representative sample[126], so most Americans are under-eating potassium-rich foods. The average American's potassium intake is just over half the 4700 mg daily recommended amount. That's a very disappointing statistic.

The fact that potassium helps with blood pressure reduction is something that has been studied quite a bit. In fact, studies on the effects of potassium on high blood pressure go way back to the early part of the twentieth century. A researcher named Addison experimented at the time on patients and on himself. He saw the blood pressure lowering effects of potassium administration in the body and concluded that high blood pressure was the result of low potassium in the diet, in conjunction with excessive sodium intake[127,128]. What is clear is that adequate daily (and I emphasise *daily*) intake is necessary to control high blood pressure. The blood pressure lowering effects of potassium are not limited only to individuals with hypertension; even those lucky people with normal blood pressure can benefit from the positive effects of potassium[129].

The effect of potassium on blood pressure occurs in a linear fashion. The more potassium you have in your diet, the higher the effect on your blood pressure readings. It's a linear, dose-response effect with potassium consumption[129]. And what's the estimated dose in relation to blood pressure reduction, you ask? You should expect a reduction of 1 mmHg in systolic readings and a 0.52 mmHg reduction in the diastolic readings for every 600 mg of potassium that you consume per day[129]. This is independent of your starting potassium level for any given day.

If you manage to meet the 4700 mg target for the day, you should expect an average 8 mmHg systolic reduction and a 4.1 mmHg reduction in readings. This is, however, dependent on race and your relative consumption of other minerals like sodium, calcium, and magnesium. Black people should expect a greater reduction in blood pressure with potassium consumption[127]. Match all of this with a reduction in sodium intake and you should find a decent reward in your blood pressure readings.

Could you have a short cut by using potassium supplements? Maybe but the results do not compare with getting your potassium from your diet. A review from the Cochrane

Database looked at high quality scientific trials that used strict inclusion criteria. The review found no significant effect of potassium supplementation on blood pressure reduction although suggested further trials that are longer to reach a firm conclusion[130].

The point there is not everything that is provided by nature can be substituted with the reductionist principle of supplementation. In plain English, supplements are not always a direct substitute for natural nutrients. I never ever advise anyone to take potassium supplements because their safety margin is too narrow for my liking to recommend their use to anyone. If you have significant kidney disease, especially those with chronic kidney disease stages 3, 4 and 5, this warning is even more imperative to steer clear of potassium supplements. The main reason is excessive levels of potassium can lead to abnormal electrical impulses in the heart. This will result in abnormal heart rhythms which can be potentially fatal.

Below are some foods rich in potassium for you to include in your diet and boost your potassium intake.

Food	Potassium Content per 1 cup (mg)
Beet greens (cooked)	1309
Raisins	1228
Prunes	1276
White beans (cooked)	1004
Lima beans (cooked)	970
Swiss chard (cooked)	962
Yam (cooked)	911
Banana (1 medium)	902

Food	Potassium Content per 1 cup (mg)
Spinach (cooked)	840
Avocados	728
Split Peas (cooked)	710
Plantain (cooked)	663
Fat free yogurt (plain)	625
Sweet potatoes (cooked)	572
Mushrooms (Portabella cooked)	529
Pomegranate juice 100%	533
Tomatoes (canned)	528
Cantaloupe	473
Grapefruit	416
Apricots	401
Coconut water (fresh)	396
Fat-free dairy milk	366
Mandarin orange	324

Source: USDA indicates the United States Department of Agriculture

Bottom line is this: get your potassium from potassium-rich foods, not from supplements.

Foods Rich in Magnesium

Magnesium was another nutrient reported to be under-consumed by Americans by the Dietary Guidelines for Americans report[125]. Americans consume only a third of their recommended daily allowance. Epidemiological and

experimental studies have demonstrated an inverse relationship between magnesium levels and blood pressure. Small
changes in magnesium levels influence how stiff or relaxed a
blood vessel is[131].

My personal experience of using magnesium over two
decades in obstetric patients with severe high blood pressure from a condition we call pre-eclampsia convinces me
that magnesium does have blood pressure lowering effects.
Yes, we use it in combination with other blood pressure medications in severe pre-eclampsia, but arterial relaxation and
increase in blood flow is usually apparent following administration of magnesium sulphate. Women always report a feeling of warmth and feeling flushed once magnesium has been
administered. This effect is due to the blood vessels becoming
relaxed, leading to an increase in blood flow.

So, how does magnesium work to lower blood pressure?
Magnesium lowers the amount of sodium inside our cells, as
well as the amount of calcium. Magnesium is a natural calcium
channel blocker[132]. It does the kind of job Big Pharma medications like amlodipine and nifedipine are designed to do.
Magnesium also stops sodium from doing a nasty job when it
attaches itself to the smooth muscle that gives our arteries their
strength and pliability. More importantly, magnesium works
in tandem with potassium in a co-operative, synergistic way to
exert its blood pressure lowering effects[129,133]. What this means
is that trying to boost one without the other is not a smart idea.
Ideally, you want to increase magnesium and potassium levels
simultaneously in order to achieve better blood pressure control, and this works even better if you combine it with dietary
sodium reduction.

One study[134], albeit small, showed modest blood pressure reduction in uncomplicated hypertensive patients. The
researchers administered 600 mg of magnesium per day to

one half of the forty-eight hypertensive patients recruited, and these patients were also given lifestyle advice. The other half were given lifestyle advice only. The study ran over twelve weeks and ambulatory blood pressure monitoring (my favourite blood pressure monitoring method) was used. The researchers found a 5.6 mmHg reduction in systolic blood pressure and a 2.7 mmHg reduction in diastolic blood pressure in the group given magnesium, while the control group had a 1.3 mmHg reduction in systolic blood pressure and 2.4 mmHg reduction in diastolic blood pressure. Reductions in blood pressure in the magnesium group occurred over a 24-hour period, so both night-time and daytime blood pressure were affected by the magnesium therapy. Not only this, but the researchers confirmed a reduction in the content of sodium and calcium inside the cells.

So, what foods can you eat to get adequate magnesium? Here are my favourite foods for boosting magnesium:

- Dark chocolate (90% or more)
- Cacao powder
- Soybeans
- Spinach
- Swiss chard
- Hemp seeds
- Lima beans
- Buckwheat
- Oats
- Wholegrain cornmeal
- Navy beans
- Pumpkin seeds
- Brazil nuts
- Almond nuts
- Peanuts

- Black beans
- Tofu
- Pinto beans
- Chickpeas
- Cooked tempeh
- Tuna
- Brown rice
- Avocados
- Bananas

Foods High in Nitrate

In the late 1980s, researchers were discovering something new. It was advanced research that turned what was initially thought to be a poisonous molecule into something that would have a huge impact on cardiovascular health in humans. A lot of work had been going on in the field of immunology and neuroscience during this time, and this fortuitously dovetailed into the cardiovascular system. The molecule in question is nitric oxide, a powerful smooth muscle relaxant with potent blood pressure lowering effects. For their efforts, three gentlemen, Robert Furchgott, Louis Ignarro, and Ferid Murad, received and shared the Nobel Price for Physiology and Medicine in 1998. Brilliant! If anyone ever tries to downplay the effects of nitric oxide on blood pressure, just remind them of that pedigree. It got three individuals a Nobel Prize, and that's not something you can just dismiss.

So, how do you get nitric oxide into our body to ignite its effects? It's simple. Eat nitrate-rich foods. And there are plenty of nitrate-rich foods about. How you eat them doesn't matter so much.

Case in point: I was someone who relegated vegetable and fruit smoothies to the background. This was because I felt the mileage of nitric oxide from the smoothie was less than eating them in the salad format. But I have since changed my mind.

Here is what I mean. When you chew a nitrate-rich vegetable like spinach in the form of a salad, you allow the saliva and bacteria in your mouth to mix with the vegetable by the mere fact of chewing thoroughly. In the mouth, there is an enzyme called nitrate reductase which converts the nitrate in the vegetable to nitrite.

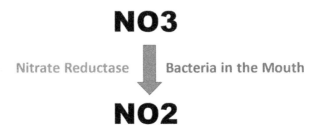

Figure 8

In the stomach and the smaller intestines, the nitrite is further reduced to nitric oxide which is subsequently absorbed. This reduction of nitrite to nitric oxide is facilitated by the acidity of the stomach. The process is also boosted by vitamin C and other polyphenols because they are reducing agents too. Just another reason why you should consume antioxidant-rich foods.

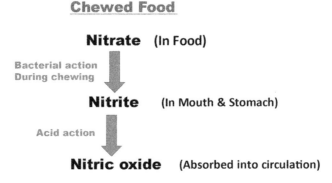

Figure 9

The process of conversion is not a fool-proof experience. Some of the nitrates are not converted to nitrites in the mouth and some of the nitrites don't get converted to nitric oxide in the stomach and beyond. Meaning we have residual nitrates and nitrites. These residual nitrites and nitrates are absorbed as they are into the blood circulation where they are recycled through the process again. About a quarter of the circulating nitrates in the blood are taken up by the salivary gland from the circulation.

These nitrates trapped by the salivary gland are concentrated more than tenfold by the gland and released in the saliva[135]. Then the previous reaction takes place again. The nitrate reductase enzyme found at the back of the tongue converts these residual recirculated nitrates into nitrites in the mouth. The nitrite is then further reduced to nitric oxide (NO). About three-quarters of the absorbed nitrate is lost in urine with only about a quarter being trapped by the salivary gland. This translates to a lot of nitrate wastage.

That process I have described above is what we refer to as entero-salivary circulation and is shown below.

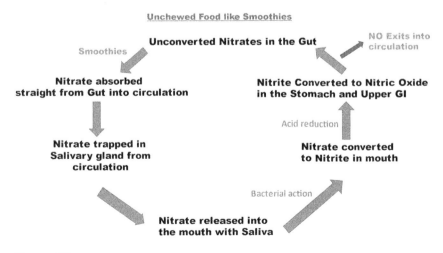

Figure 10

Above is the diagrammatic description of how we get our nitric oxide from our foods containing nitrates.

A word of caution. Some animal foods do contain nitrates. However, you do not want to access your nitrates from animal sources in particular processed meats. This is because the nitrates available in meats are prone to being converted to nitrosamines which are potentially carcinogenic. What we want to do is get our nitrates from plant sources and cash in on the entero-salivary circulation to boost our nitric oxide levels in the body.

My reluctance over smoothies initially was based on the absence of chewing as smoothies are basically drunk without chewing. So, you miss out on the initial nitrate reductase reduction of the nitrates before the smoothie hits the stomach. All is not lost though because we can still get some nitric oxide from the absorbed intact nitrates which will be re-circulated through the salivary gland and saliva. Hence, I changed my mind and now use smoothies again for my blood pressure control instead of relying on salads only. There is a lot of chewing involved with salads. And when you are doing this chewing every day, it can become a bit of a chore. Although a chore that's worth having. But having vegetable and fruit smoothies as part of the nitrate boosting plan does soften the blow. If there is any reason why we insist you have vegetables in your diet if you want to control your blood pressure naturally, it is because of nitric oxide benefits. Of course, vegetables have other benefits, inclusive of antioxidants too.

Something else you need learn here is to stop killing the bacteria in your mouth by using mouthwash. You need the bacteria in your mouth to provide you with the nitrate reductase enzyme. Without it, that conversion won't take place. Just brush your teeth as usual – no follow-up with mouthwash is required if you want to preserve your mouth bacteria. Nitric oxide production in the body declines as we get older[136]. This is particularly true if you do not take active steps to boost its presence. Natural production of nitric oxide declines by as much as 50% when we advance past the age of 40. The point here is that younger folks may turn up their noses at nitrate-rich foods like vegetables and may do all right without them. However, older folks need a little help in that department, and should be actively recruiting nitrate-rich foods into their diet to boost health, athletic performance and, more specifically, to lower blood pressure.

Making nitric oxide is one thing, utilising it is quite another though. I shall talk about that concept in the exercise chapter, but for now, you can get started with making the nitric oxide first. Why do we need nitric oxide then? Because nitric oxide is one of the most powerful smooth muscle relaxants around today. It's the discovery of the beneficial effects of nitric oxide that got those three scientists the Nobel Prize. Your blood vessel wall is made up of smooth muscle, and if you relax that smooth muscle, you increase the elasticity and pliability of the arteries, which lowers blood pressure. Eating nitrate-rich foods is therefore the beginning of wisdom if you are hypertensive.

Here are some nitrate-rich foods for you:

- Beetroot
- Spinach
- Arugula (wild rocket)
- Parsley
- Radishes
- Turnip
- Celery
- Swiss chard
- Chinese cabbage
- Leeks

- Lettuce
- Fennel
- Kale
- Watercress

One study[137] recruited forty-five healthy young men aged 18–40 with normal blood pressure and gave them a nitrate-rich juice to see the effects on their blood pressure, amongst other outcome measures. This group were compared to another group, who were given a nitrate-poor juice. The researchers found that the nitrate-rich juice was able to reduce diastolic blood pressure. Remember these are people with normal blood pressures right from the onset. The notion that nitrate-rich foods help people lower high blood pressure is a fact and an easy lifestyle measure you can easily incorporate.

Beetroot Juice

It would be remiss of me to write a sub-chapter about nitrate-rich foods and ignore the wonderful effects of beetroot juice, otherwise known as beet juice. This juice has been extensively studied and usually delivers results in terms of athletic performance and cardiovascular effects in the form of lowering blood pressure. Indeed, beetroot is the vegetable with arguably the highest nitrate content.

It has to deliver results if it's going to be the poster boy of nitrate-rich foods. One four-week, placebo-controlled, double-blind study[138] recruited sixty-eight people with hypertension aged 18–85 and gave them 250 ml of beetroot juice or a placebo beetroot juice. Blood pressure was monitored daily by patients at home for the four weeks, followed by a two-week washout period during which blood pressure monitoring was continued. Ambulatory blood pressure monitoring was also used in the study, and on each visit to the research centre, blood pressure was measured again.

Clinic visit blood pressure readings showed a reduction of systolic blood pressure by an average of 7.7 mmHg and diastolic reduction of 2.4 mmHg. Ambulatory blood pressure monitoring (my favourite) showed a reduction of 7.7 mmHg systolic and 5.2 mmHg diastolic. Home monitoring blood pressure readings improved as the experiment progressed, with peak decreases in blood pressure reaching 8.1 mmHg systolic and 3.8 mmHg diastolic. Remember the amount used in the study: participants consumed 250 ml, or 8.5 oz.

One meta-analysis[139] pooled twenty-two beetroot studies together and found a consistent blood pressure reduction. The analysis also found a greater reduction in blood pressure the longer the participants used beetroot juice, as well as a dose-related response. Higher amounts of beetroot juice gave a greater reduction in blood pressure. So, there you go. Beetroot juice is certainly one thing you can introduce as an additional weapon in your arsenal for natural blood pressure reduction.

Prescription

Regardless of the diet you choose, having a wider selection and inclusion of foods high in antioxidants, potassium, magnesium, and nitrates should be your utmost priority. Eat a variety of these foods daily and consistently and it will pay off in your blood pressure readings.

A short cut to using these foods to lower your blood pressure is to have a green smoothie at least five times a week. Stuff green vegetables with a high nitrate content into your high-speed blender, add one or two fruits to sweeten the smoothie, blend and enjoy a blissful drink that will heal you in more ways than one. As a guide, your blender jar should be 80% full of high nitrate veggies, and 20% made up of fruit. An extra step will be to add one or two tablespoonful of ground flaxseed into the mix before blending to provide some Omega 3 fatty acids. Remember I talked about blood pressure reduction being one of the benefits of Omega 3 fatty acids. Here is one unmissable opportunity to get them into your dietary plan.

If you're not into smoothies (and you should be, by the way), then have a big bowl (and I mean a *big* bowl) of salad, of which the bulk is high nitrate greens, and sweeten it with some fruit and a healthy salad dressing. Enjoy!

I'd like to add here that this prescription is more or less mandatory. Yes, I know you don't like being given orders, but this is one instance in which you will need to make an exception. Dr Joe says to do the above, without fail. And do it at least five times a week. You want to lower your blood pressure, don't you?

CHAPTER 12

What About Salt?

If there is one nutrient that has generated controversy in the last hundred years or so, it has got to be salt. Whilst some salt is needed for good health, it is by no means a nutrient that should be consumed ad libitum. But the lure of profits has provided the motivation for some corporate bodies to pull the wool over our eyes regarding salt consumption.

I'm looking at you the Salt Institute and EUsalt. These two bodies have done their best to feed the public with messages that can only be likened to what the tobacco industry did in the 1940s, 1950s, 1960s and even the 1970s. Both bodies have promoted studies that encourage the use of salt without setting adequate warnings in place to the unsuspecting public. As karma would have it the Salt Institute has shut its doors. EUsalt is still thriving though.

Whilst writing this book, I did a little search on the EUsalt website[140]. They claim to be responsible for meeting 77% of the world's salt requirements and you would think the known dangers of salt overconsumption would flash somewhere on their resourceful online platform. I entered keywords like "heart attack", "kidney disease", "stroke", "high blood pressure", "hypertension" into their knowledge database. Guess what happened? Not one search returned any results. They are essentially telling us that those dangers of eating too much salt do not exist regardless of the amount consumed. A body like that has a responsibility to warn the public about the dangers of salt overconsumption, but they don't. Better to bury bad news about salt and make it look as though it is the most innocent looking substance available to man.

I'm not the only one mad at these two institutions, Michael F. Jacobson, Ph.D., co-founder, and executive director of the Center for Science in the Public Interest is just as unimpressed and aggrieved. He said this about the Salt Institute:

"Over the years the Salt Institute has purposefully muddied the waters on sodium intake and health, going as far to say that Americans are eating just the right amount of sodium, a position rejected by virtually every health authority."[141]

That's right. Muddy the waters, confuse the public and let the trend of salt overconsumption continue. After all, salt overconsumption is good for profits, right? That's exactly what the Salt Institute and EUsalt have done over the years. A later paper extolling the virtues of salt and its safety was one published in the Lancet[142] in 2018. It was an epidemiological study involving 95,767 people in eighteen different communities. The researchers used the quantity of sodium and potassium the participants excreted in their urine as a surrogate marker for estimating sodium consumption. This is fair, considering how difficult it is to estimate actual salt intake given that consumption is spread throughout the day and that salt is hidden here and there in different foods.

They found no association between sodium intake and adverse cardiovascular events when consumption was between 4.43–5.08 g per day. There was a strong association with strokes when the mean sodium intake was 5.58 g per day. The researchers did admit that there was a systolic blood pressure increase of 2.86 for every 1 g mean increase in sodium intake, and this was seen more in those who were consuming higher amounts, presumably above 5 g per day. I'm glad they admitted that higher consumption of sodium was associated with an increase in blood pressure, even if their threshold was higher. The researchers concluded that we should only be worried if sodium intake exceeds 5 g per day. Sodium consumption below 5 g per day should be considered harmless, according to them. It is these kinds of research findings that encourage people to continue with their current levels of salt consumption. A quick trip to my local supermarket revealed why salt intake is way off the charts in the general population.

Here is what I found by simply picking a few products off the shelves at random:

Product	Amount of Salt Per 100 gm
A can of chopped tomatoes	300 mg
A tin of mackerel	910 mg
Chilli cooking sauce	790 mg
Roasted salted peanuts	700 mg
Tomato puree	500 mg
Cracker biscuits	1,300 mg
Soy sauce	1,900 mg
Barbecue sauce	1,200 mg
Rice pudding	110 mg

I avoided looking at a lot of the obvious salty foods like the canned soups, canned legumes and vegetables, chips (crisps), cereals, pasta sauces, sandwiches, sausages and ready meals, all of which are consumed daily and often.

How about fast foods? Subway, the fast-food restaurant, has handed us a digital chart of their menu, so we can have a look when we feel like it. This is good because I *did* have a look[143].

Here are a couple of Subway foods and their salt content per serving:

Food	Amount of Sodium in mg Per Serving
Veggie patty	573
Steak melt (with mozzarella cheese)	676
Cheesy garlic toastie	737
Tuna and mayo	520
Roast beef	510
Chicken teriyaki	712
Chicken and bacon ranch melt	985
Smashed falafel	911
Italian BMT (with salami, pepperoni and leg ham)	1010
Buffalo chicken	1100

That's just a handful of some of the foods on their menu. Apart from fruit juices and fruit purees, there was not a single food on the Subway menu with sodium levels below 100 mg per serving. Is it any wonder we have problems controlling high blood pressure in the community? Salt is everywhere – and I mean everywhere. People are consuming between 9–12 g of salt per day[144]. Yes, really!

This is happening despite the World Health Organisation (WHO) recommending we minimise our salt consumption to 5 g per day. That's the equivalent of 2 g of sodium per day[144].

For simplicity, this is around one teaspoon of salt per day; one teaspoon of salt is actually 2.3 g of sodium to be precise. By the way, the terms "salt" and "sodium" can be somewhat confusing as per weight. For avoidance of doubt, 40% of salt is made up of sodium. So, 5 g (5,000 mg) of salt for instance contains 2 g (2,000 mg) of sodium.

The American Heart Association's recommendation is in line with the WHO's salt prescription: no more than 2.3 g (2300 mg) of sodium per day. An ideal target would be 1.5 g (1500 mg), and for those with high blood pressure to limit their sodium consumption to 1 g (1000 mg) of sodium per day[145]. The reason for these limits is that we have ample research showing a strong association between increased salt intake and adverse cardiovascular outcomes, including an effect on blood pressure.

There is a meta-analysis[146] that looked at 133 separate studies. Yes, you read that right: 133 studies pooled together and analysed. Every 50 mmol reduction in urinary salt excretion (which correlates with consumption) resulted in a 1.1 mmHg drop in systolic blood pressure and a 0.33 drop in diastolic blood pressure. This effect was seen across diverse populations, and the older the participants were, the higher the effect on their blood pressure. This means that older folks experienced bigger blood pressure reductions when they reduced their salt intake. Additionally, non-white populations saw bigger reductions in their blood pressure for every inch of salt reduced, and if an individual's systolic blood pressure was higher from the onset, they also saw bigger decreases in their blood pressure. A dose-response effect was the order of the day. The more salt that was cut out, the bigger the reduction in blood pressure, especially in the population subsets mentioned earlier on – older folks, black people, and those with higher starting blood pressure.

Now have you ever wondered why the salt industry is highly protective of their product despite its relative affordability in the open market? Salt is quite cheap off the shelves, but the industry still manages to keep their books in the black regardless. Yes, there is household consumption, but this alone does not explain the relative financial buoyancy of the salt companies. The bulk of the profits of the salt industry come from the widespread use of salt in the fast-food industry. The fast-food industry is a more profitable client of the salt industry than regular households. One main ingredient that makes your fast food so palatable is salt and salt is also one ingredient that explains our addiction to those fast foods. All of that translates to repeated consumption of those foods, and better turnover for the salt companies. Another point to note is that food preservation requires the use of salt and the meat industry in particular relies heavily on salt to preserve the shelf life of their product. Hence the meat industry represents another demand point that makes the salt industry commercially viable come rain or shine.

It is clear there are two schools of thought here. The pro-salt group who believes you need more and more salt. And, of course, those of us who believe salt reduction is the way to go. Both sides are deeply entrenched in their positions, and this has been acknowledged. A consensus meeting was called sometime in 2018 involving both sides of the argument, to see how we could bring an end to the salt wars[147]. The Institute of Medicine, the World Heart Federation, the European Society of Hypertension, and the European Public Health Association all agreed that randomised controlled trials have become necessary to settle the differences between the two sides. Such randomised trials should have cardiovascular events, stroke, and mortality as outcome measures. This is due to the fact that all the salt research studies to date have been of a population-based trial format. The studies have been largely epidemiological as opposed to randomised controlled trials.

The problem, though, is the practicality of conducting randomised controlled trials in a free society. Such a study would be difficult to sustain by participants in the medium to long term. Adhering to a daily 1800–2300 mg sodium intake has been shown to be difficult for trial participants to stick to for longer than six months. That's the reality of salt trials; to get the true picture and an indisputable result, we need "controlled environments". A suggestion has therefore been made to conduct a trial using prison inmates. It is easier to enact such a trial in this kind of setting because of how prison food is prepared. The salt content in prison foods can be controlled with certainty, but then again, there will be other variables to correct for in a population of prison inmates, such as exercise and other lifestyle issues like drug misuse, which are painfully rife in prisons. In the meantime though, we still have plenty of evidence – albeit epidemiological – to suggest that uncontrolled salt consumption is contributing to high blood pressure, stroke, heart attacks and, of course, death. The evidence may not be of the highest quality, but the correlation is convincing enough to advise salt reduction.

By the way, the emphasis here is on reduction of consumption. This is not a no-salt approach. Our bodies need sodium as a mineral to function properly; sodium is a necessity. Having no sodium intake is equally as dangerous as overconsumption. It is about finding that sweet spot, which is one of the questions that should be answered in any proposed randomised controlled trial. Restricting consumption to between 1500–2300 mg of sodium would be a reasonable thing to do, and I endorse this wholeheartedly.

So, how do you judge how much salt is in the food you are buying at the supermarket? Below is a little guide for you,

courtesy of Action on Salt[148]. Read the food label to see what
category the food you are buying falls under.

Salt Amount Per 100 gm of the Food	Salt Content Category
< 0.30 g (300 mg) of salt	Low
Between 0.30–1.5 gm (300–1500 mg)	Moderate
More than 1.5 gm (> 1500 mg)	High

My suggested approach for salt reduction:

Do not eliminate all salt from your food in one fell swoop.
You won't like the taste of your food. Cardboard, anyone?
You'll feel disappointed and will quickly go back to old habits.

Instead, opt for a gradual reduction in your salt intake. The
beauty of human nature is that our body's systems can and
do adapt very easily. One such adaptable system is your taste
buds. Your taste buds are shed every twenty-one days or so,
meaning your new taste buds will gradually get used to your
new salt preferences. Remember that we are not cutting out all
salt; we're just aiming for a reasonable reduction.

Here is something else: when your taste buds adapt to your
new salt regime, you will appreciate the depth of salt concentration the next time you consume inflammatory foods loaded
with salt. I had a personal experience a while back when my
sons bought me a pizza because they wanted me to relax my
healthy-eating rules for "one night only". This was nice of them,
but every bite of that pizza felt as though I had scooped a tea-
spoonful of salt into my mouth. Every bite. Why was that? It was
because my taste buds had adapted and moved on from such
a heavy salt overload. If you ate those foods on a regular basis,
though, you would never appreciate the saltiness in all its glory.

Here is a bonus taste benefit for you: reducing your salt
intake also makes you appreciate the flavours of your herbs

and spices even more. Using herbs and spices to compensate for less salt helps immensely.

I have just provided you with a guide on salt labelling in food above. Please read food labels and shop smartly.

Steer clear of canned vegetables with added salt. For instance, buy canned chickpeas in water rather in salt water. Anything labelled "in brine" means "in salt". Same difference.

Use condiments (herbs and spices) to add flavour to your food. This enables you to use less salt overall when cooking.

Salted peanuts, salted cashew nuts, salted pistachios taste heavenly. That much I can confirm. Tasty but they are only boosting your salt intake further. These aren't good for your blood pressure even though nuts are good for you. Go for unsalted nuts and seeds when shopping.

If you are one of those people who will add salt to food even before tasting it, it's probably about time you dropped the habit. Have a nice taste of the food first and you might just enjoy your meal without adding more salt.

Be on the lookout for foods with the highest salt content. Here are some to become aware of. Practically most processed foods like:

- Baked beans
- Soups
- Ready meals
- Restaurant meals
- Sauces like soy sauce, BBQ sauces
- Processed meat such as ham, sausages and bacon
- Salad dressings
- Smoked foods like smoked mackerel, smoked salmon
- Fast foods like McDonalds, KFC, Subway, Pizza Hut, Domino's Pizza
- Takeaway or takeout foods

- Some cereals
- Your bread is not immune from salt

Prescription

You saw from the preceding chapter that increasing potassium intake whilst reducing sodium intake works in tandem for blood pressure reduction. This is true. You want to do both for optimal results: increase your potassium intake and peg down your sodium intake.

How about increasing your consumption of fruits and vegetables whilst gradually squeezing out your favourite salty foods simultaneously? That's how you beat this thing called hypertension, folks. Little steps like these.

CHAPTER 13

Herbs and Spices for Blood Pressure Control

Herbs and spices represent the nexus where orthodox medicine either overlaps or conflicts with traditional complementary medicine. I did mention in the preceding chapter about how practically most Big Pharma medications have their origin in plants. Very few medications have their origin as laboratory synthetic creations or from animal products. Most medications have roots rooted in plants. Pun intended.

Is there anything wrong with going directly to the source? Not really. Yes, okay, Big Pharma medications have quite a lot of research and development going into their formulations before they become qualitative healing entities. A lot of developed drugs never see the light of day; they either fail at the first hurdle or fail in the clinical trial phases. They may fail efficacy scrutiny when tested on animals or humans, or they may pass the efficacy test only to fall flat on their face with an intolerable side effect profile. Some lucky or unlucky drugs (depending on the way you look at it) make it to the market only to be withdrawn when new life-threatening side effects begin to rear their ugly heads, giving regulatory authorities no choice than to have them withdrawn from the market forthwith. First do no harm, right?

The trajectory of travel of drug development can sometimes be unpredictable. For instance, some drugs end up in unforeseen destinations. Not geographically speaking, but in terms of final clinical uses. Some drugs end up with additional clinical uses that were not previously conceived, and a few others wind up with a complete re-positioning of their use. A case in point here is Viagra. If there was ever a drug that had pulled in so much money in such a short amount of time for a Big Pharma company, Viagra would have very few competing with it. A drug that has made Pfizer billions of dollars, and still makes multiples of millions a year, is not to be sneered at.

But this was a happy accident from Pfizer's point of view. Viagra was developed by Peter Dunn and Albert Wood, and I am not making the last name of the second gentleman up. With a surname like that, he was destined to come up with a discovery like this. The original concept was to develop a medication for high blood pressure and angina, a condition in which your chest becomes tight because of reduced blood flow to the heart muscle. In clinical trials, they decided to try the drug on men who had been working in the mines in South Wales, United Kingdom. The choice to use these miners was not necessarily for blood pressure control evaluation; Pfizer wanted to assess whether better blood flow in the lungs of the miners would be feasible from using Viagra. After all, widening blood vessels was the original concept of the drug in the first place; it didn't matter in which organ the improved flow occurred.

What happened next is what Pfizer would call a stroke of luck, or serendipity might be a better word for it. The miners experienced a side effect that they loved; waking up in the morning in your 50s or 60s with a nice morning glory is not something any man would complain about. Ask any ageing man and they will confirm this. This happened across the board, and did I hear Pfizer say "ka-chin"? Let's just say that ageing men today aren't complaining either. In fact, they have never been happier. I regret not buying Pfizer shares in early 1998; that's all I'll say.

Now, let's come back down to earth, as I have digressed hugely. That being said, if you have high blood pressure, relaxing funny stories should be a part of your life. You need to chill; you need to relax. Relaxation is good for your blood pressure. The point is this: if Big Pharma can get their wallets lined using plants, you could also get those herbs and spices to work for you for next to no financial cost. There are quite a number of herbs and spices you can turn to for your blood pressure control, some of which are scientifically tested, others not so much. I talked about the meeting point between modern medicine and traditional complementary medicine, and that meeting point is where research enlightens us on the effectiveness of these herbs and spices, and also elaborates on their safety profile. We don't want to sail blindly into the alley of traditional complementary medicine; that would be fool hardy. We want to be sure our herbs and spices work to reduce blood pressure and that they are safe for us to enjoy without concerns.

Now let's have a look at some of the herbs and spices that fit this agenda.

Hibiscus Flower

The hibiscus plant is a tropical plant, a really beautiful thing to behold. The flowers are just glorious to look at any time of the day but are most beautiful on a sunny morning. If you live in a place with tropical weather, I would encourage you to have a couple of these gorgeous plants in your front garden.

The hibiscus flower will give you a bit of relaxing pick-me-up positivity every morning; a perfect start to your day.

Beyond their natural beauty, this gift of nature has medicinal properties too. Known botanically as *hibiscus sabdariffa*, this plant has been studied extensively. Many of these studies are geared in the direction of its use for blood pressure control. One such study[149] looked at hypertensive patients aged 30–70 years of age, who were randomised to receive hibiscus tea or placebo over a six-week period. Blood pressure was measured at the beginning of the study and weekly. Hibiscus flower tea was shown to reduce systolic blood pressure by 7 mmHg and diastolic blood pressure by 3 mmHg when compared to placebo.

Another study[150] put hibiscus head-to-head with captopril blood pressure medication. The captopril arm of the study received 25 mg of captopril twice a day and the hibiscus arm received tea amounting to 10 g of anthocyanins daily before breakfast. The study ran over a four-week period, and results showed that hibiscus reduced systolic blood pressure from 139 mmHg to 123 mmHg and diastolic blood pressure from 90 mmHg to 79 mmHg. What's more, captopril did not perform better than hibiscus. Those included in the study were aged 30–80, and none had been on any high blood pressure medications for at least a month.

Can hibiscus tea help individuals with a combination of high blood pressure and type 2 diabetes? One study[151] suggests that yes, it can. An average of 22 mmHg point reduction in systolic blood pressure was seen in study participants who consumed hibiscus tea compared to those who consumed black tea. In fact, the black tea caused a rise in blood pressure. The study participants had mild hypertension and type 2 diabetes and were not on any blood pressure medication or blood lipid lowering medication.

How does hibiscus flower tea work then? It is thought that the antioxidant effects of the anthocyanins in the hibiscus flower help with blood lipids with a knock-on effect on atherosclerosis[152]. That's one mode of action, but a more plausible explanation is its effect on sodium expulsion from the body, or what we call natriuresis[150]. It is thought that the phytochemicals in the hibiscus flower encourage our kidneys to reduce reabsorption of sodium, leading to a high sodium excretion. Reduced sodium reabsorption in the kidneys shrinks blood volume and consequently lowers blood pressure. This latter mode of action is more immediate than the former; the former is more of a medium to long term effect.

One thing to note with hibiscus use is this: to see therapeutic benefits, consumption should be in the region of three to five cups per day. Drinking the tea just once per day is considered under-dosing and will not move the needle for you. This is what several studies have revealed and is my own personal experience too.

Ginger

You see ginger root in most kitchens. Both fresh and dried versions. What most people do not know is that ginger is useful for blood pressure management. Most people are familiar with the use of ginger in morning sickness but its application as an herb goes beyond that. The active ingredient in ginger that helps with blood pressure management is gingerol. Gingerol is believed to act as a calcium channel blocker[153], which is the same way medications like amlodipine and nifedipine work. Seeing as gingerol appears to have the same mode of action, if you are using calcium channel blocker medications you want to be careful when consuming ginger alongside your medications.

Ginger is not only good for blood pressure control, but also helps with the prevention of high blood pressure. One population-based study[154] involving 4,628 individuals found that those who consumed between 2–4 g of ginger per day had a lower risk of developing hypertension, meaning that consuming ginger on a regular basis is a good lifestyle measure for hypertension prevention.

And what about using ginger as a herbal remedy for high blood pressure? A systematic review[155] found that using 3 g or more of ginger caused an average reduction of systolic blood pressure by six points and a diastolic reduction of two points. Adding ginger to your diet, or consuming raw ginger in tea format, wouldn't be a bad move if you have hypertension.

Cardamom

A nice spice for your food but you could get more from it. Cardamom has blood pressure reducing characteristics. A twelve-week study[156] for twenty individuals with stage 1 hypertension given 3 g of cardamom in two divided doses found a reduction of both systolic and diastolic blood pressure over the three months of the study. The cardamom also made the blood of the participants thinner as shown in the participant's blood tests. Cardamom reduces blood pressure by blocking calcium channels and also making you pee more just like the thiazide blood pressure medications.

Thyme

There are no human studies to date to support recommending thyme as a blood pressure reducing agent. I felt I should mention it here, though, because animal experiments have shown that rosmarinic acid (which thyme has in abundance) can influence your blood pressure. Rosmarinic acid has been demonstrated to exhibit anti-inflammatory, antioxidative and tumour-inhibiting characteristics in animal experiments[157].

If you remember the chapter in which I discussed kidney function and how it impacts our blood pressure, I mentioned the angiotensin converting enzyme (ACE), which converts angiotensin 1 to angiotensin 2. Angiotensin 2 is a very powerful blood vessel narrowing biological molecule. Anything that blocks the activity of ACE is a good thing for your blood pressure; it's what medications like ramipril, captopril and lisinopril are designed to do. Rosmarinic acid in thyme has been shown to reduce ACE activity by 55%[158]. Would this have an effect on blood pressure? Logically speaking, yes, and these folks' experiments on rats prove this[159].

So, despite the fact that there haven't been any trials on humans, including thyme in your diet on a regular basis is an idea worth implementing.

Parsley

I would theorise that parsley is one herb that is grossly under-utilised in the West. We are therefore missing out on the benefits of this awesome plant. Parsley is blessed with antioxidants in the form of vitamin C and several carotenoids. Antioxidants prevent free radicals from oxidising cell constituents and lipids like LDL cholesterol. Oxidised molecules and cell components are harmful to health, and antioxidants are our generous electron donors. Remember them?

Parsley has plenty of these antioxidants. In an animal experiment, hypertensive rats and rats with normal blood pressure were given extracts of parsley over a seven-day period[160]. The researchers found a reduction in blood pressure in both the rats with normal blood pressure and the rats with hypertension.

Both systolic and diastolic blood pressure were lowered in both sets of rats.

Yes, I know it was an animal experiment, but I would encourage you to start including parsley in your lifestyle. Both curly-leaf parsley and flat-leaf parsley. In fact, I will go as far as saying stop using parsley as a garnish. Use it as a main vegetable ingredient in your cooking instead. Also endeavour to use it in your smoothies too. You'll be glad you did.

Basil

Another herb that graces our kitchen countertop every now and again is basil. You may want to start using this herb to add flavour to your meals more often, knowing that it does more than bring quintessential aromatic flavouring. Basil has been in use in Asia – or more specifically, in China – for centuries. Known botanically as *ocimum basilicum,* the Chinese have always seen this herb as a cardiovascular disease remedy. An animal experiment of basil in rats showed a reduction of both systolic and diastolic blood pressure by 20 mmHg and 15 mmHg respectively[161]. Captopril did a better job in the rats, though, reducing systolic and diastolic blood pressure by 35 mmHg and 22 mmHg respectively.

In another rat experiment[162], an extract from the basil plant was found to have a blood vessel relaxing effect on the arteries, inhibiting the contractions of the arterial walls. In addition, the extract was shown to reduce platelet aggregation by as much as 53%. This is a finding re-echoed by other scientists who are investigating the usefulness of basil[163]. This feature is very important, as it stops your blood from becoming too sticky. Basil has a polypropanoid compound in the form of eugenol. This polyphenol is thought to block calcium channels too, thereby inducing arterial wall relaxation.

As a bonus for you, the polypropanoid eugenol can also be found in cloves, cinnamon and nutmeg[164].

Cat's Claw

Cat's claw is another plant quite popular in Oriental medicine. Various phytochemicals have been extracted from cat's claw, and a typical example is geissoschizine methyl ether. Hirsutine and gou-teng are also cat's claw derivative extracts. These phytochemicals have been extracted and experimented on animals. What has been found is that gou-teng, for instance, works through the nitric oxide pathway to relax blood vessels[165]. Geissoschizine methyl ether works through the calcium channel blocking pathway[166]. There are various species of cat's claw, with varying effects on blood pressure.

Hawthorn

Hailing from the Rosaceae family of plants, hawthorn is another plant that the Oriental population have used specifically for the treatment of hypertension. Hawthorn is blessed with procyanidins and flavonoids, which are both powerful antioxidants. Some of the flavonoids in hawthorn include vitexin, luteolin and rutin. These flavonoids have particularly robust blood vessel widening capabilities and were shown in one animal experiment to improve coronary blood flow (blood flow to the heart muscle)[167]. The mode of action of hawthorn seems to be through the nitric oxide pathway, just like some of the active ingredients in cat's claw[168].

Celery

I have a personal fondness for this wonderful plant. For those of you who are familiar with my YouTube channel, you will

know that I have done a couple of videos on celery. I have bene-
fited from using its juice, and I have encouraged my viewers to
use it too. Since discovering the benefits of celery for my health,
I have never looked back. Also known as *apium graveolens*, this
is a plant that is blessed with magnesium, potassium and a
phytonutrient called 3-N-butyl phthalide. Together, these phytonutrients work synergistically to produce a blood pressure
lowering effect.

Many studies have been conducted on celery seeds, presumably because of the convenience of acquiring seeds and
their reduced bulkiness. In one experiment, N-butyl phthalide
was shown to halt the progression of advanced kidney disease
in rats[169]. A six-week study using celery extract at a dose of 150
mg per day and supplying 85% 3-N butyl phthalide showed
an 8 mmHg drop in systolic readings and a similar 8 mmHg
reduction in diastolic readings at the six-week mark[170]. This
research further confirms the calming effects of celery on the
heart by slowing down heart rate and widening blood vessels
through calcium channel blocking activity[171].

One question that kept arising from the celery juice video was
whether a smoothie version would have the same effect. I was
initially reluctant to give the green light on using a smoothie
in place of juice, however I have lately changed my mind on
the issue. I had a two-month run on using a celery smoothie
while totally excluding the juice. My results were the same as
with the juice, and since then, I have switched to using a celery
smoothie 65% of the time and having the juice 35% of the time.
My initial reluctance was based on the amount of celery that is
used per session. With the juice, you need 16 oz (500 ml). To get
these 16 oz, you need two bunches of celery. With the smoothie,
I struggled to get in eight sticks of celery, which meant using
less, which was not acceptable to me at the time. However, my

testing revealed that eight sticks of celery is enough to get similar results as those you might obtain with the juice.

I have since gone one step further in making things better for myself by purchasing a high-speed blender with a bigger smoothie jar capacity. I now have a 1.5 litre smoothie jar, which means I can now fit a whole bunch of celery into my smoothie. Brilliant!

You can do the same, and even if you don't, aim to squeeze in at least eight sticks of celery and you should still do all right. Now, not everyone will like the taste of a pure celery smoothie. But what to do in this instance is simple: sweeten your celery with fruits. I have experimented with all sorts of fruits, from bananas to mangoes to strawberries to kiwis to apples to watermelon. I have had a lot of fun doing fruit experimentation, and sometimes having more than one type of fruit gives the smoothie an even better taste.

Simply experiment with different fruits to see where your preference lies. Having several recipes with different fruits also prevents boredom. As for the celery juice, you do not need fruit to go with it; drink it as it is. One reason I am leaning more towards the side of the smoothie lately is because the flavonoids within the celery are bound to the fibre, which is discarded as pulp when you juice. I think that's a vital loss, which can be avoided with the smoothie. Having said that, the juice still works regardless.

There's one more thing about celery: people get all hung up about its salt content. I can reassure you that it isn't a problem; I have tested this objectively when I did my celery juice seven-day run. I tested my blood electrolytes at the beginning of the seven-day run, the morning before I started the run and after the seven-day run. What happened to my blood sodium levels? There was no change. No change at all.

Our bodies are intelligent. Your body knows the difference between added salt and natural salt; your body may struggle to deal with added salt, but it knows what to do with natural salt. Your homeostatic mechanisms will kick in and take care of any presumed excess sodium from celery. For me, celery is just one wonderful plant you must use often, if not every day, for your blood pressure management. Use celery in one form or another, that's my big tip.

Moringa

Africa and, arguably, the Indian subcontinent have a fantastic magnitude of UV radiation from tropical sunlight. This means that plants can thrive easily so long as there are no disruptions to their natural water supply, such as drought events. Sadly, the continent of Africa also carries its fair share of environmental microbes, but plants are known to be very adaptive.

In keeping with this characteristic, plants in Africa have had to develop chemo-protective phytochemicals. You need to have the right weapons in place to protect yourself if your environment is hostile, and it isn't just humans who do this – plants do too, and very well at that. These weapons that plants have are the antioxidants I told you about in earlier chapters.

The more challenging the environment is, the more defensive weapons a plant develops and deploys when necessary. Plants in Africa and in tropical environments, therefore, have a superior nutritional profile, as well as a superior pharmaceutical profile. This is in comparison to plants grown in the northern hemisphere; it's just the way it is. It's a natural phenomenon at work, which we humans can exploit if we want to. There are apparently 45,000 species of plants (not just moringa) in Africa, of which 5,000 are used for traditional medicinal purposes[172,173]. African biodiversity can help the West.

Moringa is a plant that's been used both in Africa and the Indian subcontinent, as it grows easily in both regions. As usual, the West is late to catch on, but we are finally getting on board the moringa train. Searching through a database of research papers for publications involving moringa, there is an avalanche of scientific studies on the plant. Lots. Most of this research is on animals, which tells me that moringa has generated so much interest over the past couple of years that the hunt is on for verification of what moringa can or cannot do.

One thing is clear: moringa has lots of potential uses. Its effect on blood sugar which, in effect, ties it to diabetes management is something that will be a talking point in the years to come. Watch this space.

Let's turn our attention, then, to high blood pressure and moringa.

Phytochemicals like a thiocarbamate glycoside called niaziminin and isothiocyanate glycosides have been isolated from the leaves and seeds of moringa. All of these extracts have been found to have a calming effect on the cardiovascular system – on the heart and the blood vessels – and have also shown an ability to lower blood pressure[174,175,176,177].

How does moringa work to lower blood pressure then? The suggestion is that it stimulates the nitric oxide release pathway[178]. That said, a laboratory test showed that the molecule niaziminin from moringa blocks the ACE enzyme from doing its job, meaning moringa works like an ACE inhibitor, just like ramipril, lisinopril, and captopril. Besides, a 10 g serving of moringa powder has 160 mg of potassium and remember that we are always looking for ways to get our potassium levels up. Moringa is clearly a decent source of this mineral; I am loving this plant more and more.

Sadly, there haven't been many high-quality human studies evaluating the effects of moringa on blood pressure to date, but I did my own experimentation two years ago. I am always up for being the guinea pig for products once I am convinced about laboratory findings[179].

My personal experience with moringa is well documented on my YouTube channel. I did a seven-day run on moringa to test drive it two years ago, and I had a wonderful time with it. Moringa is like celery to me; I love both plants. My blood pressure lowering results were good. I did say in the video that I was still eating healthily, and did my daily exercise, both of which would have contributed to my awesome results. I used moringa powder at the time and still do. I am confined to using moringa powder as I do not live in an environment in which I could have a moringa plant in my back garden. The moringa plant doesn't survive frost, so if I planted it where I live, I may obtain some leaves in summer only for the plant to be killed off during the winter months.

On the other hand, if unlike me you live in a place where the weather is favourable, please get this moringa plant and cultivate it. I say that because the medicinal properties from the fresh leaves will be superior to the dried powder that most of us in the northern hemisphere have access to.

Green Tea

This is another tea that has been extensively evaluated over the years. Practically every man and his dog want to know if this magic tea from the East actually does what it says on the tin. There is an avalanche of studies in the database of publications regarding green tea and, to a lesser extent, black tea.

The essential difference between green tea and black tea is their fermentation and oxidation. Black tea is fermented and oxidised, whereas green tea is not. Oolong tea is somewhere in the middle: partially fermented. Otherwise, all three herbal teas (green tea, black tea, and oolong tea) come from the same plant by the name of *camelia sinensis*. The way they are processed is what makes the difference between them.

With all the studies available, it is not easy to make any sense of the true effect of green tea on blood pressure scientifically, because the findings are somewhat conflicting. Some studies show blood pressure reducing potential, and others not so much. In fact, there are studies that suggest an increase in blood pressure when study participants consumed green tea, and black tea is even worse. Lots more studies show that black tea does increase blood pressure, although not by a huge margin. The reason is that black tea, by virtue of being oxidised, has more caffeine extracted per unit volume of the *camelia sinensis* plant.

This study[180] that recruited individuals with high normal blood pressure or mild systolic hypertension in the range of 130–150 mmHg is a case in point. The study participants were made to drink green tea or black tea. They drank five cups a day. Blood pressure was monitored by the ambulatory method. At thirty minutes, green tea raised systolic blood pressure (top reading) by 5.5 mmHg and diastolic blood pressure (bottom reading) by 3.1 mmHg. Black tea was worse raising systolic reading by 10.7 mmHg and diastolic by 5.1 mmHg average for the study participants. This was an acute response to the tea. Over the 24-hour period, the blood pressure raising effect of both black and the green tea gradually became attenuated. But there was still an increase of 1.7 mmHg systolic and 0.9 mmHg diastolic for green tea. For black tea, an increase of 0.7 mmHg systolic and decrease of 0.7 mmHg diastolic.

A meta-analysis of ten trials with 834 participants showed that green tea, or black tea, has the capability to reduce systolic blood pressure by 2.3 mmHg and diastolic blood pressure by 1.7 mmHg in individuals with prehypertension and those with frank hypertension[181]. If you isolate the active ingredient in green tea and give it to obese hypertensive women, the effect of blood pressure reduction is the same. When a green tea extract was given to a cohort of obese hypertensive women, an average of a 3.6 mmHg reduction in systolic readings and a 1.2 mmHg drop in diastolic readings was demonstrated in comparison to placebo[182]. A slightly lower reduction in both systolic and diastolic blood pressure readings was noted at night-time. The difference between daytime and night-time could be shown because ambulatory blood pressure monitoring was employed in the study.

Why, then, are there so many conflicting results with green and black tea? In all honesty, I am not surprised at this situation. Let me explain why. You might remember that I touched on this very issue when I discussed caffeine in coffee in an earlier chapter.

Green tea has a fairly potent antioxidant called epigallocatechin gallate, otherwise known as EGCG. This polyphenol has been studied intensely, and as I write there are more studies being carried out about the applications of this biological molecule from the green tea plant, *camelia sinensis*, in particular its use in cancer prevention and treatment.

Whilst this research is underway, what we do know is that epigallocatechin gallate (EGCG) has the potential to reduce blood pressure. That's what antioxidants do, because antioxidants have the ability to widen blood vessels, thereby lowering blood pressure. That's an established fact, but we also know that the green tea plant carries the baggage of caffeine too, and that can be a problem because caffeine is a drug. A drug that stiffens blood vessels following consumption. I was therefore not surprised to see green tea and black tea studies that found a rise in blood pressure during scientific trials.

We have a scenario here where the parent plant, *camelia sinensis*, has a phytochemical with the ability to lower blood pressure, and another phytochemical with the opposite and opposing characteristic of raising blood pressure. Which of these phytochemicals wins is dependent on individuals and their genetic make-up. I do not want to go over the mechanics of how your genetics play a role in this event. If you want to know more about it, please go back to the chapter on coffee and caffeine for a reminder. It all relates to whether you are a fast caffeine metabolizer or a slow metabolizer. Of course, another small matter related to this is your sensitivity to caffeine. The more sensitive you are to caffeine, the higher the likelihood a blood pressure rise will occur when you drink green tea, black tea or oolong tea.

How individuals respond to these teas will vary, and by the way, this includes matcha tea, which is also a direct product of the green tea plant. My advice has always been this: if you are going to use green tea for blood pressure manipulation purposes, only use decaffeinated green tea. It's a safer bet and, just like hibiscus tea, positive results will only be achieved when you drink three to five cups a day. The same applies to black tea, oolong tea and matcha tea. If you can lay your hands on the decaffeinated versions, it's best to use those. But if you consider yourself a fast caffeine metabolizer and you are caffeine *insensitive*, then you may use the regular green tea, black tea, oolong tea, or even matcha tea.

Cacao Powder and Cacao Nibs

This is one of my favourite foods to have for blood pressure control purposes and improvement of general health. I know the word "superfood" is bandied around these days for everything under the sun, but this label is befitting of cacao powder and cacao nibs. Cacao powder and cacao nibs come from a plant called *theobroma cacao*. This plant produces cocoa pods from which cocoa beans are harvested. One common question has always surrounded the difference between cocoa powder and cacao powder.

I shall answer it here briefly. Here is what happens in the cocoa industry: when the beans are harvested from the cocoa pod, they are air-dried to reduce their moisture content. Subsequently, the cocoa beans are loaded into a pressing machine, which squeezes out the oil from the beans. This oil is the cocoa butter that you are all too familiar with, and this cocoa butter is put to different uses, including skincare products. What is left of the dried cocoa beans after they have had the butter cold pressed out of them is either pulverised into powder form or chopped into tiny pieces. The tiny pieces of the dried and cold-pressed cocoa beans are sold as cacao nibs. If these are ground up into powder form, you wind up with cacao powder.

The product on this end of the spectrum is a healthier one, as there is very little processing involved and nutrients are preserved. That's cacao powder. However, food manufacturers always want more, and they love processing foods to the hilt. Some batches of the cocoa beans are left to ferment and are heated to varying temperatures. The beans are roasted, so to speak. Not only this, but the beans are also alkalised – a process referred to as Dutch processing. These roasted, Dutch-processed beans are ground up to make the cocoa powder you know and love. Of course, there's a spectrum of processing in the making of cocoa products, meaning adding sugar, dairy and all sorts of additives and preservatives. This is how you get a lot of the tasty chocolate products you see on your supermarket shelves. The point is, the further down the production line a cacao bean slides, the unhealthier the final product is.

So, the difference between cacao powder and cocoa powder is that cacao powder is unprocessed (it is simply dried, and the butter is squeezed out from the beans) but cocoa powder is processed (fermented, roasted and alkalised). Your tasty chocolates are even more heavily processed. To put it another way, cacao powder and cacao nibs are wholly natural, whereas cocoa powder isn't.

What difference, then, does processing have on the final product? A lot, actually. The more processing the cacao bean undergoes, the higher the magnitude of the loss of micronutrients. The micronutrients that concern us here are the antioxidants (mainly epicatechins) that should help us to reduce our blood pressure. Roasting the cacao beans and Dutch processing them progressively reduces the antioxidant content of the cacao beans[183,184]. A loss of epicatechins in our cacao beans renders the product ineffective for blood pressure reducing purposes.

What effect does cacao powder have on blood pressure? My belief in the effectiveness of cacao in lowering blood pressure comes mainly from the research endeavours of the folks at Brigham and Women's Hospital hypertension group. These guys wanted an answer to the question of whether there were protective genes against developing hypertension, and the search for an answer took them to a remote location: the offshore San Blas islands on the Caribbean Coast of Panama, inhabited by the Kuna Indians. They wanted a group of individuals who were essentially genetically in-bred and had no influence from Western civilisation. The Kuna Indians were a good fit for the study.

What stunned the researchers was how the elderly Kuna Indians had blood pressures of below 110/70 mmHg, with no exception. That is a rare thing, for there to be no exception. Was it their genes that protected them? It turned out that this wasn't the case because the Kuna Indians who had migrated to the urban mainland of Panama and had been exposed to Western lifestyle developed hypertension. Hypertension was common amongst the migrant islanders, and the incidence of hypertension also rose with age. Protective genes could therefore not be the explanation, as your genes are portable, meaning they stay with you wherever you migrate to and live.

The researchers were initially disappointed as their initial theory was blown to pieces with the migrant islanders having cardiovascular problems upon resettling. But they persisted with their research, and this was where it became painstaking detective work. If there wasn't a genetic explanation, what was the reason for the absence of hypertension in these San Blas islands? Good question.

The researchers excluded lack of stress as a possible explanation, and their attention turned to the diet of the islanders. Their diet was found to be particularly salty from a 24-hour urinary sodium excretion test. However, what became obvious after such Sherlock Holmes detective work was that the islanders consumed more than five cups of cacao drink per day. This was a habit of the islanders to make their water tasty, and it was a habit that was initiated at a very young age; they drank cacao from the weaning stage of their lives and continued this habit until they departed Mother Earth to the Great Beyond. Their estimated intake of cacao was 1880 mg per day[185]. The source of this cacao was also important; the islanders got their cacao from Columbian cocoa, which is known to be rich in flavanols and procyanidins. That was the end of the detective work. Mystery solved!

For me, this population-based study was so convincing that I had no hesitation in using it myself and in recommending cacao powder to others for blood pressure management. If you are looking for studies, there are quite a number of them supporting the blood pressure reducing benefits of cacao powder[186,187,188,189]. We know through flow-mediated studies[190] that the flavanols in cacao stimulate the nitric oxide pathway to exert blood pressure lowering capabilities.

Before I round up my TED talk on cacao, I should say this in the interest of balance: cacao inherently contains methylxanthines in the form of caffeine and theobromine[191]. Both are stimulating substances, and I wrote extensively about caffeine in an earlier chapter. Therefore, over here with cacao, we have the same problem as we have with green tea and coffee. However, I sincerely believe the flavanol effect of cacao dominates that of the methylxanthines. That said, I have had a few – and I mean *very* few – people that I have coached where I have advised them to discontinue using cacao powder because they were very sensitive to the methylxanthines. They were experiencing significant nervousness every time they had the product, which necessitated me to act. There will always be exceptions to the rule. Other than that, cacao powder and cacao nibs get a thumbs-up from me.

Garlic

The use of garlic as a herb and a spice is as old as humanity. Very popular in the Indian subcontinent, garlic's therapeutic application span from its anti-microbial effects to anti-tumour effects to blood sugar lowering effects to cardiovascular benefits. There are various studies supporting the use of garlic for hypertension, but more about that in a second.

How does garlic work? One word – allicin.

Allicin is an antioxidant made by the garlic plant to protect it from pests. Remember I talked about how we benefit from plants building up chemicals designed to protect them from environmental insults? These constitute the so-called antioxidants we so cherish and celebrate when we eat plants. Here in garlic, we have a classic example.

Built and trapped inside the cells in the garlic bulb, once the cells are disturbed physically, allicin is let loose. Ever noticed how once you start chopping garlic or crushing it, the smell begins? That's the allicin being released as the cells of the garlic are disrupted by your actions. The worst case of garlic pungency is when you have a couple of garlic cloves, and you blitz them in a blender. All hell breaks loose then; the smell of the garlic disperses and fills the air, and any room in your house that has open doors will soon fill with the smell. It's a case of "access all areas" when you blend garlic. The unique, pungent odour and, of course, the flavour in your recipes is really allicin at work. But allicin does not begin life as allicin; it begins in the form of a precursor, and therefore needs an enzyme for its production. Life begins for allicin as alliin. Alliin is converted by the alliinase enzyme into the allicin that we are familiar with, thanks to its unique odour and flavour. Allicin, once made, is fairly unstable though. It is quickly converted to sulphur compounds called diallyl disulfide and diallyl trisulfide[192].

It is these organosulfur compounds, which are by-products of allicin, that are responsible for garlic's preventative and therapeutic health benefits. For me and from my testing, raw garlic has a profound lowering effect on blood pressure. One of my formulas for raw garlic is over there on YouTube, but in brief, it involves using garlic, banana, and coconut water. The idea behind my formula is to supply you with 1,050 mg of potassium along with organosulfur compounds in one drink. The 1,050 mg of potassium is just about a quarter of your daily potassium needs, but it is a big step towards meeting your goal.

As you know, we are desperately poor at reaching our daily potassium requirements.

This formula of mine works like a charm. The only drawback, of course, is garlic breath, which can linger around you for hours. Some people do not mind a garlic aroma, while others resent it. I do make a joke that consumption of raw garlic can be used as a "contraceptive" – not in the true sense of the word, but in the fact that garlic breath may be potentially off-putting for your partner. He or she may run for the hills at any attempt at sexual initiation, simply because of your breath. The net result is sexual abstinence, which is the only contraceptive method with a zero percent failure rate; abstinence works all the time. So, your sex life may be ruined, but you will have fantastic blood pressure.

On a more serious note, raw garlic is one of the best natural blood pressure-reducing herbs available today, from my testing. It's just the drawback of the persistent garlic aroma that may result in unintended social distancing. That formula of mine works like crazy. For those who do not like banana (yes, there are people out there who hate bananas, believe it or not), you can use avocado instead. Now, if you've noticed, I have been emphasising raw garlic. The keyword here is *raw*.

Why have I been emphasising this? It's because heat renders garlic impotent; the alliinase enzyme that undertakes the alliin conversion is very heat sensitive. In fact, alliinase has shown to be destroyed within just sixty seconds of microwaving garlic[193]. I therefore have reservations in recommending garlic supplements to people. Yes, there are some studies supporting their use in blood pressure management, but there are many others that show garlic supplements do not work as well.

Here's why garlic supplements may be useless. The first is the heat sensitive nature of the alliinase enzyme. Most production of garlic supplements will involve some form of heating, which will kill off the alliinase enzyme before any organosulfur compounds are formed. No organosulfur compounds, no blood pressure reducing effects.

Secondly, to make their products acceptable, some garlic manufacturers do their best to remove the garlic's aroma. And indeed, they use this element as a marketing feature: "You can use our garlic supplements without worrying about garlic breath". Sounds attractive, right? What you don't know is that the organosulfur compounds are responsible for garlic's aroma. Remember that they are by-products of the allicin; strip them out of the product and you have just removed the most effective active ingredient in a garlic formula or supplement. Once you kill off the odour, you kill off the effectiveness too. The effectiveness of garlic for blood pressure reduction is directly proportional to how much allicin and, consequently, how much organosulfur compounds are present in the final product.

Bottom line: if you want to use garlic for your blood pressure control, use raw garlic. Period.

Supplements for High Blood Pressure

You will recall I talked about what happened when I opened up my online forum in 2020. The story was about the very first question that was asked when new members joined: what supplements can I use for high blood pressure? I hadn't done a video about this at the time because I wanted my members to implement the foundational measures of blood pressure management naturally first, before talking about supplements.

It turns out I misjudged human nature. We want short cuts; we want the easy road. The foundational lifestyle measures require work, and human beings dislike work. Human beings dislike effort. Let's pop the pill: easier, quicker. Hence the supplement industry makes multiple billions of dollars annually. This is all well and good but using supplements as your primary intervention for natural blood pressure management can only lead to one thing: disappointment. Supplements do not tackle the root cause of hypertension; they are a band aid, a wound plaster. Use them for their defining purpose: to supplement your efforts.

Studies about the effectiveness of supplements also have to be taken with a pinch of salt. Think about it: would a supplement company publish results of any study that says their supplement doesn't work? Of course, it wouldn't. Hence all supplements studies that prove a supplement works have been either sponsored by the supplement company or the company has some sort of affiliation with the researchers. No matter how tenuous, there's usually some link, and likewise studies that say something negative about a supplement are almost invariably independent. You may say that's the cynic in me speaking, but I am pretty close to the truth.

The problem with supplement companies is that the main thrust of what they seek is reductionist, meaning if sulforaphane is a good antioxidant found in broccoli (which indeed it is), a supplement company would want to extract the sulforaphane, distil it into a standalone nutrient and formulate it into a supplement. That approach may or may not work, but why is that? It's because usually, the whole is better than the sum of its parts. There are several factors that come into play in the human body when it comes to nutrient utilisation; there is usually a synergistic effect of nutrients and an inter-play of nutrients, in particular micronutrients. Each nutrient is helping another out, and when you isolate just one and the others are missing, the result may not be the same as seen when the whole plant food or herb is consumed. Does what I'm saying make sense to you now?

Hence, results from studies are mixed and conflicting in a lot of cases meaning results are not guaranteed for the most part. That being said, there is still some room to recommend one or two supplements for blood pressure control, so long as you uphold the principle I just outlined. Use supplements to supplement your efforts. Do not rely on them wholly.

Magnesium: you need about 300–400 mg daily
Coenzyme Q10: dose between 100–220 mg daily
Fish oil: more than 3 g daily
Turmeric: dose between 1300–2000 mg daily
Vitamin K2: for people who already have calcified arteries (plaques in arteries)
Grape seed extract: 300–600 mg daily
Hawthorn extract (leaf and flower): 300–600 mg daily
Taurine: 1000 mg daily

These represent my provisional list of supplements, but always remember – no results are guaranteed with supplements. A supplement that may work for you may not work for your neighbour next door.

Prescription

Focus your attention on herbs and spices and use a variety of these plants often. Include as many as possible in your lifestyle and use them in meals, such as adding moringa or ginger powder to your food on the table.

Go beyond using parsley to garnish foods; use it as a vegetable in your soups, stews, and casseroles. Add parsley or basil to your smoothies, add spices to your recipes often, and combine these spices for optimal results.

Use some of these plants as standalone foods, such as celery smoothies and celery juice. Look to have a celery smoothie at least about three times a week, and ensure the other days are left for darker smoothies with leafy greens or better still combine the leafy greens and celery. Have them every day. Add fruits to your smoothie to make it tasty; any fruit combination is fine. Drink the herbs that come in a tea format more than once a day (aim for three to five per day) and combine the teas to accommodate having as many as possible.

Use supplements to supplement your efforts, but do not rely on them to do all the heavy lifting for you because they simply can't.

CHAPTER 14

Alcohol and High Blood Pressure

This should be an interesting one. Alcohol. The most widely used recreational agent in the world. Legal. Stimulating. Relaxing. Pleasurable. Inebriating. Intoxicating. Soul destroying. A killer too.

Alcohol has a wide spectrum of effects, as you can see from the above. An agent that is an enjoyable entity can become a deadly agent in the wrong doses for prolonged periods. That's the difficulty with alcohol advice; sensible people will use it in small doses, while others will take it to lethal levels and find it addictive, such that they lose their lives because of it.

Sadly, these negative outcomes related to alcohol abuse are occurring in younger and younger age groups lately. People in their 30s and early 40s having their livers completely trashed by alcohol. There's something about alcohol that makes it so attractive to people. Teenagers cannot wait to reach the legal age so they can jump on the alcohol train. In some cases, they start drinking secretly before the legal age. They know it. We know it. The authorities know it but there isn't a lot they can do until an unfortunate event happens as a result. That's when they step in. The reason I am talking about this is that early starts to alcohol abuse is the reason liver cirrhosis is happening at a younger age these days.

Enough about that. Let's move on to the relationship between alcohol and blood pressure. Can alcohol cause high blood pressure? Yes, it can. And the word "can" is used advisedly there because the relationship between alcohol and high blood pressure is not so black and white. An example of this is the influence of gender on alcohol outcomes. Men deal with alcohol a little bit differently from women. Women have a better deal when it comes to alcohol because of body composition and the solubility of alcohol. Factors like body fat percentage, the distribution of body fat and body size come into play.

A group of researchers analysed data from the US National Health and Nutrition Examination Survey (NHANES)[194]. They wanted to compare the effect of alcohol on blood pressures, blood lipids and blood sugar on young binge drinkers and non-binge drinkers aged 18–45. These individuals had no prior history of cardiovascular disease. Binge drinking was defined as having more than five drinks per drinking session. They split the cohorts of individuals into those who binge drank more than twelve times per year, those who binge drank one to twelve times per year and those who did not partake in binge drinking at all.

The researchers controlled for physical activity and diet. What they found was the men in the cohort who binge drank had higher systolic blood pressure and higher total cholesterol. The women who binge drank were not affected, and neither were the non-binge drinkers. Not to be left out though, binge-drinking women had higher blood sugar profiles compared to their male counterparts. This research tells us that the frequency of alcohol consumption does have a greater impact on your blood pressure and lipid profile if you are of the male species and are in a younger age group.

In another study involving 83,947 men and women across three races, health questionnaire responses were used to judge levels of alcohol consumption, and findings suggested a direct relationship: the more you drank, the higher your blood pressure[195]. The researchers had split the respondents into three groups: two or fewer drinks per day, three to five drinks per day, and six or more drinks per day.

Two or fewer drinks per day in women produced lower blood pressures. For the men, the effect of two or fewer drinks per day was neutral. Those who drank three or more drinks per day had higher systolic and diastolic blood pressures, and this applied to both men and women. In fact, there was a higher incidence of blood pressures of ≥ 160/95 mmHg in both genders once the level of alcohol consumption exceeded three drinks per day. It is clear that drinking just a little bit more than is necessary *habitually* puts you at risk of developing high blood pressure. What if you had a drinking habit that you were not happy with and wanted to reduce your consumption? Would curbing your alcohol consumption have any impact on your blood pressure at all?

Well, this study tells us reining in your alcohol use can impact your blood pressure positively[196]. They found out in their study that reducing alcohol consumption from two drinks or less per day did not make any difference in blood pressure results. But if you drank more than two drinks per day, the reduction in blood pressure was significant. In fact, in those who drank six or more drinks per day, the reduction in blood pressure was more impactful. What this tells us is, the more you drank, the bigger the blood pressure lowering effect upon cessation or reduction by 50%.

It would appear that a threshold exists where the effect of alcohol on blood pressure begins to take a spin in the negative direction. Mild consumption of alcohol appears to have either a neutral effect or a lowering impact on blood pressure, while moderate to heavy consumption is not blood pressure friendly.

What then is the sweet spot? Clearly it is two drinks or less per day. Three drinks per day or more is where your blood pressure begins to complain about the impact of your alcohol habit. Not only does alcohol cause a rise in blood pressure at that point, but it also makes management of high blood pressure harder to achieve. Now let us define what "a drink" is. This is important, as "a drink" might mean different things to different people. For the sake of ambiguity, let us zoom in on what this represents.

According to the National Institute on Alcohol Abuse and Alcoholism, a standard drink contains 14 g of alcohol (ethanol)[197]. If we go by this measure, one drink is:

- 12 oz of regular beer, which has about 5% alcohol
- 5 oz of wine, having usually about 12% alcohol
- 1.5 oz of distilled spirits, containing about 40% alcohol

There may be slight variations between different brands of alcohol. For instance, wines do come in different alcohol concentrations, and you may find a bottle of wine with an 8%, 10% or even 14% alcohol concentration. The higher the percentage concentration, the more alcohol there is in it. Regardless of the different alcohol concentrations in different bottles, if you remember the numbers above, that should give you a good guide on drink standardisation. In any case, most people who drink regularly tend to have their favourites, so you should work out what "a drink" is within your regular alcohol choices well ahead of time.

Now that we know that alcohol does have the potential to cause a rise in blood pressure, how does it do it? This study gave a group of participants 0.75 gm/kg of body weight alcohol diluted in orange juice[198]. The researchers measured the study participants' heart rate, blood pressure and muscle sympathetic activity using nerve conduction studies. Within thirty minutes of alcohol consumption, blood alcohol level rise was significant, but more importantly, there was also a significant increase in heart rate, blood pressure and sympathetic nerve activity. The researchers concluded that the rise in blood pressure was the direct result of an increase in sympathetic nervous activity. A similar study using three glasses of sparkling white wine containing approximately 30 g of alcohol produced similar results after twenty minutes of consumption[199]. The researchers noted that sympathetic nervous activity was revved up after twenty minutes of plying the study participants with white wine.

Now let's dig a little deeper into the cardiovascular effects of alcohol.

Alcohol causes an initial relaxation of blood vessel walls; this is the reason you feel warm and flushed at the initial stages of drinking. This may explain why consumption at low levels may cause a reduction in blood pressure, but as you drink more, this relaxation becomes reversed. A stiffening of the blood vessels dominates, and this is primarily due to the overdrive of sympathetic activity that I talked about earlier on. Secondly, alcohol is thought to have a stimulating effect on cortisol too. High cortisol levels are a recipe for poor blood pressure control. There may also be an indirect effect on the renin angiotensin aldosterone system (RAAS). Remember the RAAS?

Additionally, there is another theory that alcohol may inhibit the nitric oxide pathway[200]. We need our nitric oxide to help us to relax our blood vessels. A fourth mechanism is that alcohol causes magnesium depletion. Magnesium, as we saw in previous chapters, is pertinent to our blood pressure regulation. You need your magnesium for adequate blood pressure control and anything that interferes with the availability of magnesium or how your body utilises it is bad news for your blood pressure.

There is also an indirect effect of alcohol on blood pressure. The first thing to know here is that alcohol is high in sugar, meaning it carries some weight in terms of calories. Drinking often means consumption of these empty calories in excess causing weight gain, which translates to excess body fat. Excess body fat leads to high blood pressure. People who drink often and excessively also hardly ever exercise, which compounds the problem of weight gain. To make matters worse, heavy drinking is nearly always associated with a poor diet.

What about sleep and alcohol? Alcohol interferes with REM sleep, which is the restorative aspect of sleep. Poor quality sleep is not your friend if you have high blood pressure. Are you beginning to see how alcohol can cause high blood pressure and also make management of your blood pressure difficult? Think about it. If you drink heavily, are you likely to comply with taking your blood pressure medications? Probably not. Even if you were attempting to use lifestyle measures to control your blood pressure, would the picture of compliance with the measures be any different? Probably not.

Here is a synopsis of what I wrote on my blog regarding alcohol and blood pressure management[201]:

- Low level consumption of alcohol has only a temporary and minimal effect on blood pressure
- Low level alcohol consumption may not affect blood pressure adversely long term
- Low level drinking may have a beneficial effect on the cardiovascular system within reason
- The threshold for alcohol having a harmful effect on blood pressure is three or more drinks per day

- A drink is defined as 14 g of alcohol – see above for guidance
- Safe limits will be one drink per day for women and two drinks per day for men
- Sustained and habitual drinking of three or more drinks per day will cause high blood pressure in a normal person
- Having three or more drinks per day will make your high blood pressure worse and more difficult to manage
- High blood pressure caused by alcohol affects all races equally – white, black, Hispanics, Asians alike
- Cessation of alcohol will cause a reduction of high blood pressure
- Resumption of alcohol consumption after cessation will cause high blood pressure again
- Poor response to blood pressure pills and other lifestyle measures may be due to alcohol intake

Prescription

I do not recommend using alcohol as a means of controlling your blood pressure just because some research suggests that low-level drinking may help. However, for those individuals who feel that alcohol is mandatory in their lives, they may find consolation in the fact that low level consumption may not necessarily be a bad thing.

Be careful with your alcohol use. Spreading your drinking over a few (and I emphasise a *few*) days of the week would be a good compromise. Consider limiting your drinking to three days a week – but that doesn't mean you should binge drink to compensate for the days you aren't consuming alcohol. Please apply common sense.

CHAPTER 15

Sleep and Stress

Here's an assignment for you. If you happen to know one of those people who decided to pack it all up and move deep into the countryside, find out how his/her blood pressure is doing. You know the scenario I'm talking about: the person in question gives up the job, sells the house, sells the car(s). Uses the money to pay off all of their debts, builds him/herself a log cabin or some sort of shelter in the middle of the woods.

The idea? To live off-grid; to live off the land. To leave the stress of the city behind and give up on the usual daily grind completely. If you happen to know one of these wise folks, check his/her blood pressure. It will be perfect. You will get a perfect reading, probably in the range of 100/65 mmHg, unless they have a secondary cause of hypertension. If not, you should expect to find a perfect blood pressure reading. Why is that?

A move like that eliminates practically all of the stresses you can think of. All modern-day stress will be banished, for good, last seen in the rear-view mirror of their last car ride. The bonus is that these folks will also be eating whole foods. These will be nutrient-dense, packed full of antioxidants and all the micronutrients you can think of. There will be no concerns regarding pesticides because they grow their own food.

Check out their body composition too: less than 10% body fat, without even trying. The fat falls off them, based purely on the clean eating that is inevitable with a lifestyle like that. Plus, the absence of a car means they walk everywhere, alongside the physical activity of cultivating their own food. Plus, there are no unfriendly neighbours to worry about. The perfect life, I think. Have I sold the lifestyle well enough for you yet?

While I am not recommending that we all up sticks and pursue this way of life (although you can if you want to), a move like that proves one thing: we are all stressed. Modern life is stressful; we have worries about jobs and job security. Worries about deadlines at work. Worries about finding a suitable life partner if you are still single. Worries about mortgage payments. Worries about car payments. Worries about rent payments if you are a tenant. Worries about health. Worries about health insurance. Worries about ageing parents and their failing health. Worries about the kids, from school to university or college. Worries about online bullying. Worries about the kids making their way in life upon graduation. Worries about life after retirement. The list is endless.

Modern life is stressful. There appears to be no end to it.

Is it any surprise that high blood pressure is rampant in our society? Of course, stress alone is not the reason we are hypertensive, but it contributes to the problem, and it also negatively impacts blood pressure management. If you do not manage the stress in your life, it is going to be difficult to see blood pressure numbers on your monitor that you will be happy with. I have lumped sleep and stress management together in this chapter as both are related; in fact, they are both drivers of one another. Poor sleep promotes stress, high stress levels promote poor sleep, and the cycle continues. I will talk about sleep shortly but let me say a word or two about stress first.

Most people do not live their lives in isolation. That's aside from the folks I described earlier, who decided that living in the woods was the best thing they could do for themselves; and rightly so. But the hermit way of life is not everyone's cup of tea. Living amongst others means we have to interact in all sorts of places: at home, in the workplace, at shopping malls and airports, on airplanes, on trains, at supermarkets, on the roads. Every point of human interaction is a potential point of conflict, and all of these points are potential points of stress. If you are expecting everyone to be reasonable, then you might as well move to planet Mars. It's not going to happen, not here on planet Earth. What's weird is that even when there is no physical interaction, we can still manufacture fault lines thanks to modern technology.

There are stories of parents talking about bullying in school when they were younger. The bullying was as rampant then as it is today, but the difference is that in the 50s, 60s, 70s and 80s, there was no internet. You could be bullied at school as a young girl or boy, but at least when you got home, you knew you were safe. You were protected by your parent's shelter and love. Not anymore. Bullying today is a 24-hour source of stress, thanks to the internet. That's twenty-four hours of stress on a young mind and, of course, that rebounds on the parents too. No parent wants to see their child miserable. None.

The internet has become a lethal source of stress and it is almost inescapable. Yes, you could quit social media, but its lure is quite potent. Ever heard of celebrities shutting down their Twitter or Facebook accounts, only to be back a couple of months later? For those of us who put ourselves out there on social media and are fortunate enough to become influencers, we know we are taking a risk. Internet trolls are always on the loose, and it is difficult to rein them in. It's nice to be adored, but such adoration comes with responsibilities. That's the way I see it, anyway – others may see it differently. But there are risks too – I have been a target more times than you've had hot dinners. I'd like to think I'm a modest dude who doesn't brag about his achievements, yet I am a target just by virtue of having a noticeable social media presence. I know it comes with the territory, and one has to learn to deal with it. I'm not whining about ordeals from internet trolls but to make a point that human interactions, whether virtual or physical, are a hotspot for stress.

And the way out of it is to learn to not outsource your happiness. We are all guilty of outsourcing our happiness. I am still learning not to, I must confess. To demonstrate the point about outsourcing our happiness, imagine what happens on the road either when driving a car or riding a bike and some other driver cuts in front of you. You catch up with him at the next set of traffic lights, and the offender winds down his car window, gives you the middle finger and shouts obscenities at you, even though he is the guilty party. A scenario like that is bound to ruin the rest of your day – but only if you allow it.

Most of us will chew the event over and over again in our minds, especially when we know we were the wronged party. We will ruminate over it and allow it to dominate our thoughts for the rest of the day. What's worse is when you don't have a spontaneous comeback at the time of the argument but come up with one five minutes later when the opportunity to verbally fight back has already evaporated. *That* will annoy you to no end. Becoming upset over incidents like this is allowing someone else to dictate how you feel. That is outsourcing your happiness, and it is not good. That's just one example, but there are several others. Someone could say something unfriendly to you in the office; it could be your boss. Or it could even be your partner at home, saying something unkind to you. We, as human beings, are very good at locking remarks like that into our minds, ruminating over them and allowing them to spoil our day.

This is a classic case of outsourcing your happiness. You are letting someone else dictate whether you should be happy or sad, allowing someone else to take charge of your emotions. If they treat you well, you feel good. If they treat you badly, you feel sad. Something we have to realise as human beings is that humans are incredibly selfish; they think of themselves and themselves only. Okay, I may be making a blanket statement there – we also have people who are equally incredibly considerate – but most human beings are selfish, truth be told. Their thoughts and actions only surround themselves. How do we solve this? We must decide in advance that our happiness is our responsibility, and it should not be dependent on other people's behaviour. Quickly drawing a line under such events and moving on helps to prevent such unwanted stress.

There is the story of a popular Hollywood film director/ producer, who was absolutely brilliant at the concept of compartmentalisation. A co-producer was once at this popular film director's home. At the time, the film director was having marital issues that were all over the press. Both the film director and the co-producer were having a production meeting at the film director's lavishly furnished home. This meeting of theirs kept getting interrupted by phone calls from lawyers, his estranged wife, and other people.

The film director would excuse himself to take these phone calls, some of which lasted ten minutes or longer, and the visiting co-producer could overhear some of the heated exchanges. Not that he wanted to eavesdrop; not at all. The co-producer was not a nosey guy, but he could hear a lot. What surprised him the most was how the film director would return to the table and continue with the meeting, showing no hang-over emotions from these phone calls. Even when he had had a heated exchange over the phone just thirty seconds earlier. The film director would quickly move on and continue with his previous task. A lot of people would be unable to continue such a meeting due to the baggage from the previous phone conversation. Clearly this film director is excellent at compartmentalisation; a skill a lot of us need to acquire.

It's all about feeling happy within yourself in advance and deciding in advance that such stressful events will not bother you. Attempting to acquire this skill when the event occurs is a late intervention that won't work; you need to build it prior to the event and be ready to deploy it when needed. Everyone has a story inside them, and it's a story of contentment. Find it, sharpen it, keep it underneath your skin for easy access. Use it whenever necessary – that way you won't allow inconsiderate people to get under your skin. A friend sent me an Instagram post some time ago which I liked. These may not be the exact words, but it was something along the lines of:

"Your emotions are your personal responsibility. You decide what prevailing emotions you want to own at every minute of the day, and don't expect the world to tiptoe around you. Because it probably won't happen as you had hoped."

I couldn't have put it better myself.

What About Prolonged Stress?

The scenario I painted above is an acute stressful event, one which is supposed to be quelled by a major physiological protective mechanism that nature bestowed upon us: our fight or flight response. Nature gave us this response to use as a built-in mechanism to deal with an acute threat to our safety. That threat could be existential, in which case the system would serve us well.

A major physiological sub-event that occurs in the fight or flight response is the spontaneous release of the hormone, adrenaline. Adrenaline is a potent vasoconstrictor (an agent that narrows your arteries) and therefore increases your blood pressure. This has relevance to us as individuals with hypertension. The adrenaline surge, however, was not designed to hurt our blood pressure; rather it was designed to quicken the flow of oxygen and energy to our muscles. This prepares us for a fight if that's our choice, or flight, or both. Escape when you know the enemy is more powerful than you – after all, there is a saying that goes: he who fights and runs away lives to fight another day. Are you familiar with that saying? No? It's probably native to me, so I don't blame you if you haven't heard it before but remember it. You don't always have to be right and prove that you are. You don't need to lose everything just because you want to prove a point – even if you are right. It's most likely stressful and not worth it.

But here is the problem with millions of people all over the world. The fight or flight response, which was originally gifted to us by nature to survive immediate threats, has become a daily punitive "activity". It was designed to be a transient survival tool from threats either physical or emotional, but nature never intended for us to be in a perpetual fight or flight mode day in day out, week after week. But this, unfortunately, is the reality for most of us today. We are forever in fight or flight mode, left stranded there when the threat is long gone. Being in permanent fight or flight mode is exhausting; it's crippling. It is both emotionally and physically draining, but for most of us, it is reality. What's the outcome of being constantly in fight or flight mode? Anxiety. Depression. How severe depends on a myriad of factors, not least each individual's coping mechanism. Most of us cope poorly with the never-ending mental stimulation.

The main reason why mental aspects of life have become chaotic is because the fight or flight mode stimulates our sympathetic nervous system. Such sympathetic overdrive is never a good thing; it raises blood pressure, it makes us anxious, it reinforces the stressful situation. Therefore, any solution must involve getting the antagonist of the sympathetic nervous system to kick into gear. Enter the parasympathetic nervous system, probably one of the best natural tools you can have in your arsenal to deal with stress and anxiety. Now, let's talk about how we can call upon the parasympathetic nervous system to come to our aid.

Breathing

One automatic physiological event that occurs from the minute we are born is breathing. In fact, breathing activity starts inside the womb. Yes, babies in the womb breathe; they don't breathe in air until they are born, but they do breathe all the same. Obstetricians like me see these breathing movements on an ultrasound scan. We have to breathe to survive; it is automatic. You cannot stop yourself from breathing. Did you know that you cannot euthanise yourself by simply stopping breathing? It is impossible. Nature has checks in place to stop that from happening. If that's the case then, why don't we exploit this inevitable physiological process to the maximum for stress relief purposes – in particular, for anxiety?

Makes sense, right? After all, breathing is free. You don't have to pay for it. All you need is a little bit of time to learn how to breathe to relieve stress and anxiety. Learn the technique, perfect it, and get ready to roll it out when you need it.

And guess what? Getting your breathing technique right is one of the quickest ways to lower your blood pressure. You can use it in an emergency when stressed as, of course, your blood pressure will be high during times of stress. If a blood pressure spike is due to stress and anxiety in an acute situation, calling on your breathing technique is the quickest way to dampen the situation and get your blood pressure under control pronto. How do you breathe to lower your blood pressure then? Well, there are various techniques, and it doesn't matter which one you call upon. Just use one. Now let's talk about some of them for your convenience.

Box Breathing

You may use the box breathing technique. This one involves inhaling slowly through your nose for four seconds. Hold your breath for four seconds after inhaling slowly for four seconds. Relax your shoulders whilst doing this. Breathe out through your mouth slowly for four seconds. Pursing your lips or resting your tongue behind your upper jaw incisor teeth such that you let out the air slowly and gently making a whooshing sound helps release the exhaled air gently. Hold your breath for another four seconds (do not inhale for four seconds). Now repeat the process again. It is called box breathing in the sense that your breathing, in this instance, is shaped like a box of equal four sides. Four seconds in, hold four seconds, four seconds out, hold a further four seconds – 4 x 4 x 4 x 4. Do this several times. You will gradually see your muscles relaxing and your anxiety getting relieved.

You don't have to limit the technique to four seconds. You could do six seconds or even eight seconds in a box manner, so long as you can handle the breath-holding for that long. Do that for five minutes or longer if you wish.

Alternate Nostril Breathing

You choose how long you want to hold your breath for: four seconds, six seconds etc. You can apply the box breathing technique here. The only difference is you use your right index finger to block off your right nostril and inhale slowly through your left nostril for four or six seconds. Hold your breath again for four or six seconds. Now swap over to the other nostril blocking off your left nostril with your left index finger. Breathe out through your right nostril slowly for four or six seconds. Hold your breath again for another four or six seconds. So, you breathe in through one nostril and out with the other alternately.

Repeat the process over and over again for about five minutes. Use this method any time of the day to reduce your blood pressure and there is research evidence to support its effectiveness in reducing blood pressure[202].

Triangular Breathing

This one is also called the 4 x 7 x 8 breathing. It is simple to do. Place your tongue against the back of your upper incisor teeth and gently exhale all the air from your lungs making that whooshing sound. Expel as much air as possible as if you are completely emptying your lungs of air. Now inhale through your nose slowly for four seconds. Hold your breath for seven seconds. Then exhale gently as previously described for eight seconds.

If you have difficulty holding your breath for seven seconds, you can do triangular breathing using the four second approach instead. Breathe in for four seconds, hold for four seconds and exhale for four seconds duration. It still works. The point here is that triangular breathing doesn't have to be 4 x 7 x 8, it can also be 4 x 4 x 4 too. Either way, it is still a triangle.

Belly Breathing

Here is another one that works a treat, and you can employ it in any situation in which you are becoming stressed. You know, events like public speaking when you are waiting to go on stage, or when you are waiting to meet a new date. Once you have noticed that you are getting stressed, call on your belly breathing for emergency salvation.

A good place to start is to learn this breathing technique from babies, if you have one. Watch a baby breathe. Babies breathe through their bellies. Babies do not do chest breathing. Babies have perfected the art of abdominal breathing. It's natural for them. Quite how we transformed from that form of breathing to chest breathing is difficult to work out. Either way that transformation is totally unhelpful.

Chest breathing is inefficient. We only use a small capacity of our lungs when we do chest breathing. Belly breathing (abdominal breathing) however increases our lung capacity by at least 50%. You should be working the diaphragm muscle when you breathe. The diaphragm muscle is what separates the chest cavity from the abdominal cavity. Learn to work this muscle. You might not be able to do belly breathing all the time, because we are so accustomed to chest breathing. Why change the habit of a lifetime, eh? What we can do though, is learn belly breathing and deploy it when the occasion demands it.

So, how do you learn abdominal breathing?

Most gurus will tell you to place one hand on your belly and another hand on your chest whilst lying down on your back. Then breathe such that the hand on the belly should rise higher than the chest hand. That's one technique but I don't like that technique.

The technique I prefer is the one where you lie flat on your back of course. Place a book on your belly. Not a heavy book. A light book. Then inhale fully and watch the book rise and fall. If the book is not rising appreciably, then you are still engaging in the old habit of chest breathing. Learn to push that book all the way up whilst filling your lungs with air. One way of knowing that you are chest breathing rather than belly breathing is the movement of your shoulders. If your shoulders are rising when you inhale, you are chest breathing. In belly breathing, the shoulders barely move and 90% of the breathing movement is concentrated in your belly.

Now, belly breathe in slowly for four or six seconds. Hold your breath for four or six seconds, then gradually exhale slowly for eight seconds and watch the book lowering itself as you exhale. Practise this for around five minutes or longer each time. Once you get the hang of it, do it as a stress- or anxiety-busting technique about three to four times a day. That's how it will become a habit, but don't take it for granted. It requires practice, practice, and more practice.

There are many more breathing techniques, but if you engage with the four I have just described, you should be fine. The net objective of breathing exercises is to slow down your breathing rate and to deepen your breath. There are devices on the market that can help you with these breathing exercises; some of them are quite expensive but there are apps – some of them free too – that can assist you with learning to breathe slower and deeper. I do not want to name any such apps, as I would be promoting them inadvertently; just go to the app store on your phone and download any that suit you.

What we are trying to achieve with breathing exercises in whatever form is to have an over-riding parasympathetic nervous system domination over the sympathetic nervous system. This calms us down as it downregulates down level of activity in our limbic system, which in turn lowers our blood pressure.

Between inhalation and exhalation, however, one is more important than the other in helping us kick our parasympathetic nervous system into gear. Of the two, exhalation is the most important stimulant of the parasympathetic nervous system, so if you were to customise your own breathing exercises, the part you want to prolong the most is the breathing out.

The longer you prolong your exhalation, the better your results. Always remember that for any breathing exercise to work, the emphasis should be on abdominal breathing (belly breathing). Belly breathing works the diaphragm, stimulating the vagus nerve as well as enabling us to take in more oxygen per breath, which helps to deliver results[203]. Remember that the brain, which obviously controls our mind, is an oxygen-hungry organ. The brain is only 2% of our body weight; it weighs around 3 lbs but uses 20% of the oxygen you breathe in[204]. Think about that for a second; getting enough oxygen helps your brain to function to its full potential.

Learn from babies. Breathe like a baby and you will start winning the war on anxiety and hypertension.

Mindfulness and Meditation

You cannot talk about anxiety relief, breathing, parasympathetic nervous system stimulation and blood pressure control without delving into mindfulness and meditation. Indeed, combining both makes sense. This is one self-care intervention that is usually ignored by lots of people, and that included me for a long time. Once you get into meditation though, you will uncover a new bliss. It's the same principle of getting the parasympathetic nervous system to dominate the sympathetic nervous system.

When we do breathing exercises or embark on a meditation journey, we stimulate the vagus nerve. Once you succeed in recruiting and activating the vagus nerve, you will have triggered the antidote to the fight or flight response. This singular act quietens down fear and anger and calms the amygdala:

the part of the brain responsible for our basic emotions. Successfully doing this also stimulates parts of the frontal cortex, which enables us to think clearly, to become self-aware and to show consideration for other people around us and beyond. Meditation is one way of getting you back to physiological and psychological balance.

So, how about we do a little five-minute meditation. Now you must be wondering how do I meditate reading the text on this book? Good question. It's very simple: record the text I have written below and play it to yourself anytime you want to meditate. You will in effect be instructing yourself. It works. If you are not comfortable giving yourself guided meditation instructions, let your partner record it for you and simply play the audio back anytime you want to meditate.

Now, record all of the text below using any audio recording device you have. *But oh, Dr Joe, I don't have an audio recording device.* Not a problem; use WhatsApp. Record the passage below and send it to a friend or your partner, then the audio file will be in your WhatsApp forever, and you can play it back anytime. Either this, or a friend can record and send it to you on WhatsApp too. Easy.

This is important: when recording, the text must be read out slowly. *Really* slowly, in a soothing manner. You are not reading the news, so please do not record the text below as though you are a newsreader. Read it out slowly and leave gaps between sentences. I hopefully should have a video of this guided meditation on YouTube by the time this book is ready. And you can listen to that. Here's my guided meditation for you:

Find a comfortable place devoid of distractions. Sit and be comfortable. If it is necessary to shut the door, do that please. We want to be focused.

Now shut your eyes. Direct all of your attention to your breathing. Breathe in slowly and deeply. Take a deep breath in through your nose and exhale through your mouth slowly.

Remain focused and become aware of the depth and rate of your breathing. Remember to have all of your attention on your breath and nothing else. You should feel your lungs filling up, expanding when you inhale and your lungs shrinking as you exhale.

Next focus your attention on your physical self. Look out for any knots in your body. Tension spots. Willingly allow those tension areas in your body to relax. In particular drop your shoulders and let them relax. Really relaxed. Feel the tension melt away from those muscles and joints. Enjoy that feeling of relaxation. Ride that wave.

If your mind wanders off, that's normal. Don't fret over that. Redirect your mind back to what we are doing using your breath as your hook to bring your thoughts back. Focus on your breathing noting the current depth and speed of your breathing. The slower the better.

Think of a warm moment in your life. A wonderful beach vacation experience for instance. A day out that you enjoyed. A warm hug you had from a friend you cherish or a warm hug from your mother. Relive the experience and allow the warm and fuzzy feeling to be the only emotion you feel right now. No doubt a pleasant feeling running through your veins – let it run from your head to the tip of your toes.

A meditation moment is a happy moment. Allow the positive past experience to bring a smile to your face. It's okay to smile right now. Let the feeling sink in for the next few minutes.

Now imagine a light feather stroking your skin very gently starting from the tip of your right middle finger running up your forearm to your arm really slowly. It's now on your right shoulder wandering to the right side of your neck now heading up to your head and over your scalp to the left side of your neck.

Let the feather work its way gradually down your left arm to your left middle finger and back up and let it wander down the left side of your chest, the left side of your belly and over slowly on your left leg to your left big toe and back up to the lower part of your belly across to your right lower belly. Now let the feather wander down your right leg slowly all the way to your right big toe and gently back up to your belly.

Let the feather continue its journey stroking the right side of your belly slowly and gently over the right side of your chest. If the feather tickles you at any point, let out a gentle smile. Now finally let it wander over your right arm and forearm to the tip of your right index finger back to where it all started. Let the feather fall off and revel in the joy of what has just happened. Let out a smile. Enjoy the moment for a good minute.

Now take in a deep breath again, hold your breath for about five seconds and exhale gently and slowly. Do the deep breathing three more times taking in a deeper breath than the one before. Now squeeze your buttock muscles, contract your belly muscles, your arm muscles and clench your fists very tightly. Hold the contraction and the squeeze for ten seconds. Let go slowly. Take your time and gradually return yourself back to full blown consciousness and gently open your eyes when you are ready.

Hopefully, you feel refreshed after that round of meditation, and your limbic system will certainly thank you for it. Meditation succeeds when you successfully focus your attention on your breath and your breathing, but it takes time to get used to it. Do not feel discouraged if you don't succeed in your first few attempts; it takes practice. Make it a habit to meditate once a day, even if it's just for five minutes.

Your Sleep

Now, let's talk sleep. Sleep is arguably the most important biological necessity, beaten only by food and the art of eating. The phrase "rest and digest" couldn't be more apt – you need your sleep as much as you need your food.

Over the years, sleep has been ridiculed, made to look like something needed only by the lazy and the sluggish. Think sloth, the animal and you won't be wrong. In fact, politicians of the 70s and 80s viewed sleep deprivation as a symbol of strength. One popular female politician once described sleep as a "thing for wimps" and used to brag about needing no more than four hours of sleep a night. Her views about sleep were public knowledge, and I imagine the men in her ministerial cabinet who needed more than four hours of sleep must have felt belittled. Something like that would dent their confidence, no doubt.

That sleep habit (unhealthy as it was) served her well at the time though; she could function well on such little sleep. She was mentally sharp and would wrestle men down in political debates. In her later years though, she unfortunately suffered and died from dementia. Whether the accumulated sleep deprivation debts she acquired over the years contributed to the Alzheimer's disease is difficult to prove and is open to debate, but one thing science has established is an association between chronic sleep deprivation and Alzheimer's.

Yes, it's true some people can function effectively with very little sleep, but that doesn't make it a healthy habit. There could be medium- and long-term consequences. For instance, poor sleep may be the reason you are having difficulty losing that belly fat, despite your best efforts. Poor sleep may be one reason your diabetes is difficult to control. Poor sleep may the reason your sugar cravings are getting worse. Poor sleep may be a huge contributory factor to why your anxiety is uncontrollable, no matter what you do. One thing is certain: if you don't sleep long enough or well enough, your efforts to control your blood pressure will be seriously undermined. And, of course, that is very relevant to us here.

We talk about diet and exercise as being the cornerstones to good health, and sleep is usually given a bystander role as far as health is concerned. But that's an error – sleep is actually the foundation on which diet and exercise are anchored and should be built. If you pay lip service to sleep, you will pay the price somehow. In fact, whatever you are trying to achieve through diet and exercise will be harder to accomplish when sleep is chronically compromised. The younger you are, the more you think sleep is irrelevant. Yes, some of us burnt the midnight oil in an attempt to be studious especially in our high school and university days. But all of that was due to poor organisation, leaving a lot of our studies until the last minute when exams were fast approaching like a high-speed train. So, we scurried to get our acts together and, in so doing, sleeping very few hours. Socialisation was also a factor; being young is almost synonymous with partying. If you party often, you sleep less.

On graduating from college or university to settle down, one would expect a shift in behaviour and a move towards sleeping better. Sadly, lots of people have significant difficulties with sleep beyond their college days: problems with sleep initiation, problems with staying asleep. There are two main reasons I theorise as being responsible for the difficulties we experience with sleep, aside from sleep disorders, which are a separate issue altogether. The first is our fight or flight response issues, which I talked about in the preceding sub-chapter. Being trapped in a heightened state of anxiety generated by being stuck in fight or flight mode is an ingredient for sleep difficulties. You may remember I talked about the limbic system, and an important mini organ in the limbic system is the amygdala. The amygdala is our emotional brain; it is responsible for our basic emotions.

When we have overriding emotional issues that remain unresolved, the entire limbic system goes into overdrive. When your limbic system is in overdrive, it is very difficult to fall asleep easily. Being in a permanent state of fight or flight response does exactly this; it keeps our limbic system active. Your body senses danger in the fight or flight response mode and because we are neither fighting nor fleeing "the situation", the limbic system remains active. This interferes with falling asleep, and if you do fall asleep, you may have difficulty staying asleep for the number of hours you need in order to feel refreshed and invigorated.

In case you are wondering what emotional issues I am talking about, these don't have to be deep-seated issues, like post-traumatic stress disorder (PTSD). Everyday concerns, the types of which I listed previously (jobs, nuclear family, extended family, environment etc.) can stimulate the limbic system enough to keep you awake at night, and it's worse when the problem is existential. Type A and type D personalities are hardest hit, but everyone is susceptible regardless. We cannot escape our problems, so the best approach is to develop coping mechanisms well ahead of bedtime. The stress coping methods I described previously can be drawn on as solutions; quell or exit fight or flight mode in advance of going to bed.

Another main issue that contributes to us sleeping poorly is not correctly identifying our chronotypes and aligning them with our circadian rhythm. Circadian rhythm dictates when we feel sleepy and when we are awake; it's the 24-hour sleep/wake cycle. It's easier to manipulate your circadian rhythm than your chronotype. There are four chronotypes, but they fall into two broad categories. These categories are whether you are a night owl or an early bird. Night owls go to bed late (2–3 a.m.) and wake up late (9–10 a.m.). Early birds, on the other hand, go to bed early (8–9 p.m.) and wake up early (4–5 a.m.). You really cannot swap one for the other. And that is what most of us are guilty of. Mainly due to occupational demands. Sadly, we have to earn a living to survive.

This is another reason those folks living in the middle of woods with their care-free lifestyle do so much better with their health; they don't have to deal with a chronotype-circadian rhythm mismatch. They fall asleep and wake up at the time their chronotype dictates and are not forced into a chronotype dictated by their professional occupation. And yes, there is a difference. Chronotypes are biologically predetermined through the circadian clock gene PER3. One study[205] found that a shorter allele is associated with being a night owl, and a good 75% of patients with delayed sleep phase were homozygous for the short gene. Being an early bird, on the other hand, was associated with a longer allele.

Humans having different chronotypes is thought to be evolutionary, and it makes sense for this to be the case. Studies of the remaining hunter-gatherer communities have also confirmed this to be true[206]. If you think about it, everyone feeling sleepy and going to bed at the same time would be a potentially disastrous set up, wouldn't it? Nature designed us such that some people would remain alert while others got their shuteye. Otherwise, who would fend off danger when a lion approached in the wee hours of the morning? Hence there is no homogeneity in chronotype genes; someone must keep watch while others are recharging their brains with a well-earned rest.

The problem most of us have is matching our chronotype to our circadian rhythm. Whereas you can train your circadian rhythm – for instance, when you change time zones – it is difficult to train your chronotype, because chronotype is inherently a genetic issue. Attempting to train your chronotype means initiating a fight with our genes, and fighting our genes is always going to be a tussle, a big mountain to climb. Your circadian rhythm responds to environmental cues, like light and perhaps temperature, while your chronotype doesn't. This war of attrition between chronotypes and circadian rhythm is where a lot of us wind up with the sleep issues and subsequent fatigue that plague millions of people.

Night owls are forced to wake up at 6 a.m. or 7 a.m. at the latest for work purposes whereas their productivity time does not kick in until midday. I should know – I am one. Conversely, early birds may wake up and be vibrant in the morning hours, because they are morning people after all. Come 3 p.m. however, they struggle to be productive. They experience an inevitable slump around that time, but they have to continue working until 5 p.m. or even 6 p.m. Are you beginning to see the conflict here? The way our generic work schedules have been designed does not cater for our chronotypes' demands. I, for one, would personally prefer to start work at 11 a.m. with a view to finishing at 7 p.m. That would suit me really well, just as a typical early bird would rather start work at 6 a.m. and finish at 2 p.m. But this is not the way our job schedules are structured; everyone must fall in line with the generic office times.

How much sleep do we need then? There is no clear-cut scientific evidence that points to precisely how much sleep we require as adults. However, what we *do* have is a projection from sleep studies. Each sleep cycle lasts about ninety minutes, and it is anticipated that adults should fit in five sleep cycles per night in order to recharge our batteries. Five sleep cycles, each lasting ninety minutes, equals a total of 450 minutes. This equates to 7.5 hours, hence the estimated eight hours of sleep that is usually suggested as the optimal sleep duration. But anything between seven and nine hours is considered adequate.

Does your chronotype influence how long you sleep for? It shouldn't; your chronotype only determines the times of the day in which you are most suited to sleep and most suited to being productive. Your chronotype does not determine how much sleep you need; in fact, based on the way our work schedules have been set up, it turns out that most of us are sleeping and working in conflict with what our chronotype dictates. This is called social jetlag, and it has implications for our health. Social jetlag has adverse endocrine, behavioural and cardiovascular implications, and the longer your social jetlag is, the worse the effects. A social jetlag of ≥2 hours was found to cause higher cortisol levels in one study[207].

Do not listen to new sleep "gurus", who proclaim that your chronotype determines how much sleep you need. I have seen and heard them spreading this nonsense on social media, encouraging night owls to not do anything to get longer sleep duration if all you got as a night owl was three or four hours sleep a night, because that's what your chronotype deserves and gets. This is totally incorrect; a night owl would sleep longer if only they could, but work demands mean they can't. There is no evidence to suggest that some humans were programmed genetically to have only 3 hours sleep. You might get by on such miniscule amount of sleep, but it is not necessarily in your DNA hardware.

I know an individual who couldn't sleep beyond 4 a.m. no matter how much he tried. He went to bed around midnight to 1 a.m. so got only four hours sleep or even less. So, I suggested he adjusted his bedtime to an earlier time; gradually bringing his bedtime backwards until he went to bed by 9 p.m. It worked. Now he gets a good seven-hour sleep time. When readjusting the actual time you go to bed, it needs to be done gradually.

Usually, you should enact a thirty-minute adjustment at a time and let that sink in for a week or two before making another thirty-minute adjustment and letting your body acclimatise for another week. That's the approach – if you rush it, it will fail. Take your time when making changes to your bedtime. This example illustrates how we fail to recognise what our chronotype is. Not correctly identifying our chronotype means we erroneously do what may be in direct conflict with our predetermined chronotype. The end result? Sleep problems. He thought he was a night owl when in fact he was an early bird. It's a common mistake. If you are having sleep issues, your first task is to correctly identify what your chronotype is and align your sleep behaviour accordingly. Which brings me nicely to how to organise and reshape your sleep behaviour if you have difficulty with falling asleep and staying asleep.

Fixing Sleep Problems

I did mention earlier that you can manipulate your circadian rhythm, within reason. Your circadian rhythm responds to light and darkness, and you can train your circadian rhythm by adopting a fixed schedule.

Adopting a permanent bedtime and a permanent wake-up time is the first thing you need to do. Your body will love that, and sometimes, your body will love it so much that you won't need an alarm clock. Your body will know when to wake up because your internal clock will start sending circadian wake up signals to rouse you. Still, set the alarm clock just in case. I'm just making a point that your internal alarm clock will kick into gear once you develop a strict bedtime and wake-up time.

Once you wake up, expose yourself to as much light as possible. Commercially available wake-up lights are a good panacea for the darkness outside during the winter months, otherwise part your curtains to let in natural light. This would also be a good time to do some gentle exercise or, if you do workouts, this would be a great time to do one. The workout will not only give you those cardiovascular benefits but will add to your feeling of waking up and shaking up. It will get you more alert.

If you are the coffee-loving type, you may have your coffee now. I'm against coffee if you have high blood pressure, because of its effects. This is my view from scientific studies, but if you are a coffee lover regardless, then go ahead and have your coffee. The other rule about coffee and other caffeinated products is that they should not be consumed beyond 2 p.m. That's because it takes your body about six hours to get rid of the caffeine from your system, with implications beyond its immediate blood pressure raising effect.

Here is another thing about caffeine which I dislike: the effect of caffeine on sleep. Your body makes adenosine the minute you wake up from the metabolic processes going on in your body. Adenosine is what makes us feel tired and sleepy. The more adenosine we have built up as the day progresses, the sleepier we feel at night and the easier it is to fall asleep. Adenosine is your friend when it comes to sleep, and caffeine competes with adenosine. It blocks and stops adenosine from doing its job of making you fall asleep. That's why you get a pick-me-up effect when you consume your coffee, or any other caffeinated drink. Given that it takes around six hours for your body to completely rid itself of any caffeine consumed, it therefore makes sense not to drink coffee beyond 2 p.m. This is very important if you are having sleep issues.

Expose yourself to as much sunlight as possible during the day. Doing so reinforces your circadian rhythm. You are telling it: this is daytime. You are also telling the pineal gland in your brain not to make melatonin, which saves your melatonin production for night-time when darkness falls. Sunlight exposure equally sends signals to your brain to make serotonin, which improves your mood. Your brain and your internal clock need that reinforced daytime message signal to distinguish it from night-time.

If you did not engage in any exercise in the morning, then the daytime or in the early evening would be a good time to get some in. Exercise promotes sleep, so do not skip it (no pun intended).

Eat foods that promote sleep for dinner in the evenings: leafy greens, beans, almonds, pumpkin seeds, sunflower seeds, yogurt, cheese, salmon, bananas, kiwis, cherries (in particular tart cherries), chamomile tea, lemon balm tea, lavender tea etc. These foods provide the ingredients necessary for the making of the melatonin hormone, and the teas will provide a calming effect to your limbic system. We need melatonin to help us fall and stay asleep; melatonin is our sleep hormone (more like a sleep hero really).

Reduce your light exposure as the evening wears on. Start dimming the lights in your house as the evening progresses and remember that we are trying to manipulate our circadian rhythm to our advantage. Telling your internal clock, which controls your circadian rhythm, that night-time is here can only be a good thing. That way, the pineal gland in the brain will start making melatonin. Too much light confuses your pineal gland; in fact, too much light suppresses your melatonin production.

Reducing your exposure to light means changing your cell phone light emissions to night mode, too. Otherwise, stop using your cell phone altogether in the evenings or buy blue light blocking glasses to use from 7 p.m. The blue light emitted from cell phones and tablets suppresses melatonin production, as I mentioned earlier. Remember, you need your melatonin for sleep purposes.

Do activities that tell your body: its sleep time. Have a routine that wraps up the day. Some people will call it a winding-down routine. It doesn't matter what it is called. All that matters is engaging in activities that psychologically tell your mind and body; bedtime is coming soon; the day is over.

Avoid watching movies or TV programmes that get you excited; horror movies are included here. Similarly, don't read any texts that get you excited, either from physical books or from your cell phone/tablet. The same thing applies to audiobooks or podcasts that are designed to get you motivated. Night-time is the wrong time to move up the gears of motivation.

Alcohol is best avoided; it may help you to fall asleep easily but its effect on rapid eye movement sleep (REM sleep) is abysmal. You won't get restorative sleep and it is generally a bad idea to use alcohol as a sleeping agent.

Don't eat or drink too close to your bedtime to avoid having to wake up several times to visit the bathroom. Late night meals also affect your body core temperature as your revved up metabolism makes it difficult for you to have the dip in core temperature needed for staying asleep.

Now, go to bed and burn off the adenosine you've been accumulating all day. Sweet dreams!

You will have noticed that I said nothing here about the sleeping aids that are marketed as sleep messiahs, both online and offline. You don't need 99% of them. No matter how much the seller swears by them, they don't work. If they do, their effectiveness is short-lived. Save your money. The only exception I will make though is the sleep eye mask. I have it and I can confirm it helps block out residual light which reinforces the darkness your pineal gland needs for melatonin production. Sleep eye masks have my approval. Wear one when you go to bed; they are quite cheap and durable too. And lest I forget, a comfortable bed and mattress is never a bad idea for a good night sleep. Is your mattress due for a change, by the way? A mattress in constant use for the last ten years or so is crying for a change. Do not ignore the cry please. Does your mattress suit your body type? I know memory foam mattresses are all the rage right now, but they are not for everyone. They don't suit everyone. Surprise, surprise. A friend of mine tried for four months to like her new memory foam mattress that cost her an arm and a leg without success. In the end she gave up, asked for a swap and retailer was kind enough to accept her request for a swap for a relatively firmer foam. Never forget the role of a good mattress. The age and type of mattress are so easily forgotten when you are searching for answers to your sleep problems. That focal point of your bedroom is a sleep essential that is so easily underrated. Don't be a victim of that.

Prescription

Remember, good quality sleep is essential for blood pressure control. In fact, it is not just essential, it is imperative. Fix your sleep hygiene, match your chronotype with your circadian rhythm where possible, dump your worries in a marked "worry box" before you go to bed and a glorious morning awaits you after a good night's rest.

Learn to love your limbic system and, more importantly, love your brain as an organ. Calming your limbic system is key to blissful mental health, as it feeds on to your frontal cortex. Recruit and stimulate your parasympathetic nervous system in any way that you can; mindful meditation and breathing exercises are highly recommended.

One more thing: everyone gets stupid, intrusive, disturbing thoughts streaming into their minds every now and again. Everyone. It's normal and it's natural. Dr Amen talks about this concept too. He calls them automatic negative thoughts, but I prefer to slap an abrupt negative thoughts label on them, otherwise known as ANTs. I say they are abrupt because of their intrusive nature. But here's the thing: those thoughts are not true. Don't believe them. Believing these intrusive thoughts breeds negative emotions, and negative emotions lead to anxiety. Anxiety begets anxiety.

So, stop believing those unhelpful thoughts if you want to help your limbic system and your blood pressure. Smash the ANTs dead in their tracks when they intrude into your mind's space. These ANTs will show up intermittently, but they don't belong there – do not download them into your head, don't allow them to live rent-free in your mind. Move them swiftly on.

CHAPTER 16

Exercise for Blood Pressure Control

I'm going to go out on a limb here and make the following claim: "Exercise is the absolute best tool at your disposal for blood pressure management."

That claim is a hill I'm prepared to die on. I stand by that statement. Today, tomorrow, forever.

Unlike weight loss, in which you do not necessarily have to lift a finger and can still lose weight effortlessly using diet alone, blood pressure control plays to a different tune. It would be difficult to achieve consistent blood pressure lowering results without moving your body somehow. It's possible, but results will be limited. To get your blood pressure lowered, you must engage in some form of exercise. Period. No short cuts. How much exercise and what type can vary, but physical activity must be part of the blood pressure healing process. Here's the irony: even though exercise is the most important aspect of blood pressure management, this chapter about exercise is probably going to be the shortest in the book. Why? Well, let's face it. Is there anything to be said about exercise that hasn't been said and you haven't heard already? Probably not.

Exercise is not just good for blood pressure control; it is also probably the best thing you can do for the prevention too.

Case in point: there are three nurses I work with whose exercise habits I admire hugely. They exercise on a regular basis, almost every day, and they have been doing so for years. They are in their 40s and 50s, and every now and again I will challenge them to have their blood pressure checked at work. This is not ideal, and is a little cruel of me, because the workplace is the last place you want to have your blood pressure checked. We work in a fairly high-pressure environment, but when it quietens down a bit, that's when I challenge them to have their blood pressure checked.

They are not hypertensive, by the way. The reason I undertake this cruel act is to prove the point that engaging in regular physical exercise is the best way to prevent high blood pressure. These three nurses never disappoint: perfect blood pressure readings all the time in a stressful environment at work. I can almost guarantee that those blood pressure readings aren't going to change significantly, even when these three ladies get to their 70s and 80s. Any young person reading this book who is not hypertensive yet, here is a tip for you: exercise regularly and you will keep high blood pressure at bay.

Here's another story for you. There's a lady who lived a stone's throw from my house. Let's call her Lady A. Although I have since moved to a new house just a couple of blocks from my initial residence, I still run into Lady A at the supermarket every now and again. Lady A was, by definition, a neighbour of mine, and I have known her now for twenty years; she is still my distant neighbour even now. I want to talk about Lady A's mother, though. Let's call her Mother Hen. Mother Hen walked everywhere, and I mean *everywhere*. Mother Hen lives about five miles away from her daughter, Lady A, and, of course, the mother-daughter relationship is always a strong one. Not living that far away, Mother Hen visits her daughter often, at least five times a week. And guess what? Mother Hen never drove to see her daughter; she walked those five miles every single time. And then, of course, she walked another five miles back to her own residence. I did wonder initially if Mother Hen didn't own a car, but I was wrong. Mother Hen does own a car, but she hardly ever drives it. I suspect she doesn't do more than 500 miles a year in that car, because she walks everywhere. I recently asked Lady A what her mother's blood pressure was like. "Perfect," she responded. Mother Hen is in her late 70s now and is another case of physical activity preventing high blood pressure. Yes, I will admit that these cases are anecdotal, but they support my view regardless. Physical inactivity is one of the main causes of high blood pressure. It is amongst other factors, of course, but physical inactivity must take a lot of the blame.

We just don't take exercise seriously enough. As you saw in the earlier parts of this book, I was guilty of this crime for decades. When I started exercising after my initial diagnosis, I faltered hugely. Remember I said I didn't have awareness with conviction in my earlier attempts? Gaining awareness with conviction was what flipped the switch for me over a decade later. Obviously, I have "seen the light" now, and things have changed tremendously for me, such that I feel guilty if I take a day off without doing any of my routines. Yes, it is that serious for me. I have fallen in love with exercise, and I cannot see any divorce in sight – not if I can help it, anyway.

I have just given you some anecdotal reports suggesting that exercise is the best thing you can do to prevent high blood pressure, but there is also research evidence to support the view that planned physical activity in the form of *regular exercise* reduces the risk of developing hypertension by 33%[208]. Not unexpectedly, there's an inverse relationship between exercise activity and the risk of developing hypertension.

So, knowing that exercise prevents hypertension, does it work to control it if you already have it? It absolutely does. If it didn't, the American Heart Association Professional Education Committee of the Council for High Blood Pressure Research would not be recommending it for blood pressure control[209]. Neither would the latest update of the 2016 European Guidelines on cardiovascular disease prevention, and neither would the American Expert Panel[210,211]. Many professional bodies involved with hypertension guidelines have all recommended exercise as an essential part of managing blood pressure. In fact, some guidelines suggest initiating lifestyle management (of which exercise is a huge part) as a first step in managing high blood pressure with systolic readings of 140–159 mmHg and diastolic readings of 90–99 mmHg, without commencing medications in the absence of target organ damage[212].

This just shows you how much emphasis there now is on lifestyle changes. If you think about it, high blood pressure is, for the most part, a lifestyle disease. What is the point of jumping on medications when the root cause is still left untouched? How likely are you to win if you persist with old bad lifestyle habits? Is it any wonder over 60% of people still struggle with blood pressure control, despite being on medications? A sensible thing to do would be to tackle the lifestyle habits that have contributed to the problem in the first place. Of course, if there is damage already done to other organs by high blood pressure (aka target organ damage), then starting medications would be reasonable. And if your blood pressure is ≥160/100 mmHg, it would also make sense to commence medications too. But commencing blood pressure medications is not a reason to relegate lifestyle changes to the backseat. Both medications and lifestyle modifications must be executed alongside one another.

What kind of exercise should you be doing? Three words: all of it.

- Aerobic exercises
- Dynamic resistance training
- Isometric resistance training

Ideally, you want to combine all three forms of exercise. In my routines and the ones I use for my online blood pressure reduction clinics, I make sure we do all three as part of a package in every session.

Aerobic Exercises

Most exercises you are familiar with centre around aerobics, because they are the first set of exercises that will pop into your mind when you think about physical activity. Aerobics will improve your blood pressure, but you need to be consistent. So, what aerobics might you consider?

Walking

This is the simplest aerobics that anyone – and I mean anyone – can do. It's a low impact exercise, but it works well for blood pressure control regardless. It's basic human instinct to walk and is probably the first exercise you learnt to do as a human being. Why not cash in on it?

You can walk at any age. On my way to work every morning, I see a man in his 80s walking with his little backpack. I don't know how far he walks, but I presume the fact that he has a backpack suggests he's clocking decent mileage every day. The first time I saw him, about three years ago, I thought he was walking to see a friend. Then it became a regular daily event, and I usually drive past him at the same point on my route to work every morning; he was always dressed the same and always had his backpack. It became obvious to me that what he was doing was indeed an exercise activity as opposed to a leisure activity. During the winter months when it's dark in the mornings, he wears a high visibility jacket, so he can be seen. That's risk management for you right there. As you can tell, this man takes his morning exercise walk very seriously. He is in his 80s and he walks; what excuse do you have if a man in his 80s can programme walking into his daily schedule for three years and counting? Think about that for a second.

You remember my ex-neighbour's mum whom I thought didn't own a car because she walked everywhere? She walks, she has fantastic blood pressure, and she is not a 30-something year old either. She's in her 70s, she walks, and she's been walking for the twenty-one years that I've known her.

Here's another story to inspire you. On my route to work (again), I also spot a blind man who walks every morning like clockwork. I see him at the same spot every morning too, walking in the opposite direction to me, holding his white cane and using it to scan his path for obstacles, taking his time to ensure he's doing things right. And here's the thing. These two men, whom I see on my way to work at different exact locations every single day, walk regardless of the weather. Aside from heavy snowfall, they both walk whether it's raining, cold or perfect sunshine. They are not fair-weather walkers; they walk regardless of the weather, because they have programmed walking into their lifestyle. You can too. If a visually impaired man makes walking every morning a routine, I really cannot see why you too cannot indulge in this simplest of low-impact exercise.

You don't have to do the extreme walking exercises of going hiking twenty-one miles in one day. No, not at all. Start small and leave the twenty one-mile hikes for us, the experienced long-distance walkers. Here's my suggested walking plan for you if this is all new to you:

Walk half a mile a day. Do that for a week or two.
Then walk one mile a day. Do that for two weeks.
Then stretch it to two miles a day and do that for four weeks.
Then three miles, five days a week, and do that for two months.

You will see your fitness levels getting better and better. Ultimately, my plan is for you to walk five miles, five days a week. That's not all. Speed is very important too. It's not a stroll. It should be a brisk walk, and my recommended speed is three miles per hour. If you brisk walk the initial target of three miles, five days a week, each episode should last an hour. When you hit the target of five miles, five days a week, each walk should last an hour and a half.

How do you calculate your speed? Get an app that reports your average speed for every walking routine. I'm usually reluctant to name products here, as I don't want to be promoting any one over another, but I will make an exception here because of the functionality of this app. It's free to download, and I should say that I have no affiliation whatsoever with the developers of this app – I just happen to like it. The app is called Ramblr, and that's not a misspelling; there's no "e" in the word. Download it and, of course, turn it on as soon as you're about to commence your walk. Once you're done, you'll get some nice stats, including your speed, distance covered, the degree of difficulty and how many feet of ascent there were in your walk. When I coach people, I notice that practically everyone is obsessed with steps. Personally, I am not interested in steps, whether on your phone or using a step counter. I'm not impressed with steps; I am more of a "distance covered" person. For a start, those step apps on your phone or on step counters are usually way off the mark. They are incredibly inaccurate, and they overestimate a lot – sometimes by as much as 25%. I suspect they are built that way to please and motivate you.

I discount steps and focus on distance instead. That's my style. You may say: don't steps add up to miles? Yes, they do, but I have the hump with the overestimation which I find difficult to ignore. More importantly, how do I distinguish between the steps you did in the office, at the shopping mall etcetera versus your dedicated walking exercise routine? I do not want the lines between physical activity at your workplace and your dedicated exercise session blurred.

I believe a walking exercise session should be distinguishable from your steps at the supermarket, the shopping mall, the office or at home. A walking exercise should be a dedicated exercise session, and those stats should be different. This is serious business, and I want you to view it as such. Turn on your Ramblr app when you are about to do a dedicated session, and nowhere else. Then get walking; it's the easiest exercise on the planet.

Running

Now, here is a shocking confession for you: I am not a big fan of running. I know, I really shouldn't make a remark like that – I am trying to get you to exercise, so I shouldn't be negative at all. But truth be told, I dislike jogging. It's just not my thing. If you remember, earlier on in the book, I talked about how I jogged for a couple of months following my diagnosis of hypertension, then it all fell apart about three months later. One substantial reason for this was that I never enjoyed running, I simply tolerated it. The lesson here is to focus on the exercises that you like and enjoy.

I love walking. In fact, when I go hiking, I walk with my hiking group for ten hours or longer. I love it; I would rather walk for twelve hours than run for one hour. I mean it – I just love walking. But I *hate* jogging. But that's just me. You may be different. If you love running, please run, and run for your life. Okay, that sounds somewhat scary; it sounds as though you are running from a visible threat, like a lion. Let me rephrase that: run for your heart and your blood vessels. Regardless of my personal preference, jogging is a fantastic exercise for blood pressure. It really is. If you love it then do it with passion. Try to jog about five days a week; just like walking, targeting five miles for each running session is a fantastic idea.

One beautiful side effect of jogging is the "runner's high" that you get. Runner's high has been likened to the "high" of cannabis. Running induces the production of endocannabinoids in the brain. Those endocannabinoids are the substances that give runners that feeling of elation or better still that state of euphoria that's all too common with running enthusiasts. Running gives you that rush of dopamine in every session when you are done, guaranteed. That is why running can become addictive. Now that's an addiction worth having!

Other Aerobics

Other aerobics, such as swimming, basketball, table tennis, lawn tennis, squash, football (soccer), volleyball, martial arts, rope skipping (jump rope), boxing, home cycling on a static bike or road cycling are just as useful. My only problem with these other exercises is that they may be difficult to weave into one's lifestyle on a consistent basis several times a week – apart from swimming and cycling, of course.

But if there is a way in which you can incorporate any of these into your lifestyle, such that you can engage with the routine five days a week, then go for it. That's the beauty of walking and running, they are easily adoptable and adaptable. But if other aerobic exercises are your cup of tea, then please go ahead – consistently though.

Dynamic Resistance Training

Here is my personal experience. Doing aerobics was good for my blood pressure, but what gave me that final break was adding resistance training into my routine. The idea that resistance training is only for individuals trying to bulk up and build a physique like The Rock or Arnold Schwarzenegger (when he was younger) must be discarded. Yes, bodybuilders do a lot of resistance training, and yes, they do build muscle. It is undoubtedly so. But that is not our objective here, we are not trying to bulk up. We're simply doing our bit to lower our blood pressure. And yes, ladies need to do resistance training too – it's not an exclusive reserve for the male of the species. I promise the ladies reading this book that bulking up like a bodybuilder will not happen. Not with our approach anyway.

What makes the difference between bulking up building muscles and not bulking up is the weight of the load and the volume involved in the exercise routines. We are not interested in heavy lifting; we need some weights to give us resistance, of course, but not very heavy weights. Additionally, the volume of the exercises we will be undertaking for blood pressure controlling purposes is nowhere near what is needed for bodybuilding.

Twenty minutes of resistance training is enough for our blood pressure needs, especially when we combine our resistance training with aerobics. Twenty minutes resistance training plus another thirty minutes of aerobics is enough for one session. For resistance training, you either use free weights or your own body weight. Body weight resistance training is equally as effective as employing free weights. I love using my body weight for resistance training. Now let's talk about some of the dynamic resistance training you may undertake for blood pressure controlling purposes.

Squats

Doing squats, for instance, is dynamic resistance training that anyone can do (unless you have a knee issue). Squats are one example of body weight resistance training. I love squats; I do at least 160 squats a day, split between mornings and evenings. Eighty in the morning in lots of twenty reps (repetitions) per set meaning four sets of twenty reps. And another eighty in the evening. If you are going to do that many squats like me, make sure you get the technique right to protect your knees.

Briefly here is a quick description of the correct squatting technique. Your feet must be spread out to shoulder width at least. The idea being to distribute your body weight evenly over your two knees, hips, and feet. This spreads out your body weight, as opposed to concentrating it on your knees when they are close to one another. Your knees take the most impact during squats, as they undertake 90% of the shock absorption when you lower your upper body.

So, stand astride. Now bend as though you are trying to sit on an imaginary chair behind you, with your feet flat on the ground. Using the technique of sitting on an imaginary chair keeps your knees behind your toes during the squat. Naturally your knees are flexed, and so are your hips. How far down you go is up to you. Some people like to do a full squat, but I prefer to halt my squat when my knees are at a ninety-degree angle. That's when I reverse my squat and stand up again to complete one rep.

And what do you do with your arms as you go down on the squat? Some people fold theirs close to their chest, but I prefer to stretch mine out in front of me. Doing this provides a counterbalance to the simulated sitting position, and outstretched arms reduce the risk of falling down onto your bum as you bend down. Stretching your arms out also makes for another physical activity involving both arms too, that way the arms aren't just left redundant. Aim to do twenty reps of squats per set. Even if you do two sets which will equate to forty repetitions (reps) in one session, that's still a nice number to run with.

Push-Ups

Another fantastic dynamic resistance training exercise is push-ups. You should endeavour to include push-ups in your routine; shoot for at least eighty push-ups a day; forty in the morning, in two sets of twenty, and another forty in the evening. By the way, you can still arrive at forty push-ups by doing ten reps per set making a total of four sets. Ideally though, you may want to target 120 push-ups per day if you can (sixty in the morning and another sixty in the evening) – you will thank me later for this.

Moving on from squats and push-ups, using free weights is equally as good. The reason I like squats and push-ups is that they are portable meaning you can take them anywhere with you – and they're free too.

Free Weights

With weights, you will need to buy some stuff. Be it kettle bells, dumb bells, resistance bands or ankle weights, use them judiciously and increase the level of difficulty gradually. Don't rush the process. If you feel more comfortable going to the gym to use weights, that's good too, as gyms have a vast array of resistance equipment. The rule is to gradually increase your weight load and the volume that you do.

Sadly, using weights is where you are likely to suffer a sports injury. Seek professional help before undertaking a routine you are not familiar with, and at the very least, watch YouTube videos that demonstrate a correct exercise technique before jumping in. Remember, you do not need to do a lot: aim for a minimum of twenty minutes of resistance training per exercise session. If you can do more, that's even better.

Isometric Resistance Training

The new kid on the block is isometric resistance training. It's now beginning to assume some more significance as far as blood pressure reduction results go. Mean blood pressure reductions of 10 mmHg systolic and 5.8 mmHg diastolic cannot be sniffed at[211]. The message here is this: you must include isometric resistance training in your exercise routine.

In case you are wondering what isometric resistance training is, here it is. It's any exercise activity where you put a group of muscles under contractile tension and the joint involved does not move for the duration of the activity. Typically, the muscle length remains the same throughout the duration of the exercise activity. Isometric exercises are useful for building strength and endurance and, of course, blood pressure reduction as stated earlier. Although isometric exercises are useful for strength, this is a limited benefit. To garner enough strength from isometric resistance training, you'll need to do different types of these exercises, in order to strengthen different groups of muscles. Now let's talk some examples of isometric resistance training...

Yoga

Is yoga isometric resistance training? I believe it is. A lot of the exercises in yoga fall into the isometric profile, in my opinion, and most yoga sessions involve different postures, hence recruiting and isometrically contracting different muscle groups. It's the reason yoga exercises help with blood pressure reduction, in my opinion, along with the fact that yoga incorporates breathing exercises too. Pilates will also fall into this category.

Research evidence does contradict my view that yoga postures contribute to the blood pressure lowering effects of yoga in general, though. This study, which split up participants into yoga breathing only without yoga postures, and yoga breathing along *with* yoga postures found the yoga breathing only group to have a reduction in systolic blood pressure[213]. The researchers employed ambulatory blood pressure monitoring as their tool. Yes, it is true that yoga activates the parasympathetic nervous system by stimulating production of gamma amino butyric acid (GABA)[214]. Doing so calms down the sympathetic nervous system, thereby reducing systolic blood pressure in particular. Yoga proponents therefore seem to advise that the focus for yoga and hypertension should be on yoga breathing and/or meditation. I am still of the opinion that yoga postures do play a role, but then again, I am not a yoga expert.

I do not have much experience with yoga, as I haven't managed to find the time to learn yoga routines. Consequently, I cannot relay any personal experience with yoga or pilates as far as blood pressure reduction is concerned. Listen to the yoga experts who are more in favour of the breathing and meditation aspects of yoga than the postures. Are there any other isometric exercises that you can try at home? Yes, of course.

Planking

You can do either elbow planking or hand planking. Elbow planking is the most popular type. It is a form of planking in which a lot of your body weight is supported by your elbow and forearms. Of course, planking works the core abdominal muscles and the shoulders too. The hand plank is another favourite of mine, which follows the same principle and works the same muscles, but your body weight is supported by your flat palms on the floor. Side planking is another option. With elbow and hand planking, it is important you keep your back straight and engage your core muscles. Allowing your spine to dip or sag is a recipe for back injury. Keep your spine level, straight and firmly in the same position for the duration of the plank exercise.

Aim to plank for two minutes. Start small, in fifteen-seconds segments, and build it up gradually. You may be surprised to know that the current elbow plank world record at the time of writing stands at 9 hours, 30 minutes and 1 second. It is currently held by Daniel Scali. It is a feat worth mentioning in this book. He set the world record in Adelaide, Australia in August 2021. Don't ask me how he did it. I haven't the foggiest idea on how someone will plank for nine hours plus. But it puts into perspective that I'm only asking you for a two-minute plank per session in comparison. Two minutes should be a piece of cake, right?

Wall Sit

The wall sit is another isometric exercise you can employ. This is basically a squat hold; you may use a wall to support your back, or you may just sit in the air with your knees flexed at ninety degrees. Keep your arms stretched out and hold for fifteen-second segments. Do ten reps of this and later, aim to sit for a ninety-second hold.

Glute Bridge

The glute bridge works your hamstring and gluteal muscles, aka your bum muscles.

Lie on your back and flex your knees with your feet flat on the floor. Your arms should be by your side. Thrust your hips upwards, supporting your weight with your heels. Now, clench your gluteal muscles and you will automatically feel your hamstrings tighten at the same time. Hold for a good twenty seconds, keeping your hips elevated in the same position. Aim to do a two-minute hold over time.

Body Hold

Aside from improving your blood pressure, the body hold works your core muscles too. It's very simple to do, although it takes practice as you tend to feel unsteady when you start. Sit on the floor with your knees bent and feet flat on the floor. Now, stretch your arms out in front of you and lift up your legs, straightening them out. What you want to achieve is to have your body shaped like a triangle, with your arms nearly touching your shins. You may need to lean back a little to stabilise yourself. Hold for twenty seconds and do ten reps. Aim to achieve a ninety-second hold with practice.

Other isometric exercises include the handgrip, overhead hold, split squat, leg extensions and the static lunge.

Resistance training is held in such high regard that it is now being suggested as a first-line therapy for non-white individuals with high blood pressure[212]. This is mainly because the magnitude of possible reductions in blood pressure is tilted more in favour of non-whites than whites. Quite how and why that's the case I really cannot say, but that's research for you. They do come up with inexplicable findings like these.

The Nitric Oxide Dump Exercise Routine

It would be remiss of me to write a book about natural high blood pressure management and say nothing about the nitric oxide dump exercise routine. Most people who became familiar with my work on YouTube did so via their discovery of my nitric oxide dump routine.

My nitric oxide dump exercise video, I am glad to say, has garnered 3.6 million views at the time of writing. It is probably my best performing video on YouTube. Now, lots of videos on YouTube get millions of views for no good reason; some are packed with misinformation, but they still get lots of attention because of the way the YouTube algorithm works. Conversely, some great videos packed with sound health advice get very little exposure, which is really sad. The YouTube algorithm is to blame – it is only interested in answering one question: does this video make Mother Google money? Not: does this video contain good quality, lifesaving information? If we promote this video, does it get lots of clicks and do viewers watch much of the video? Meaning does it make Google money? If the answer is yes to both queries, the video gets all the help it needs to get seen by as many people as possible. The problem though is not all uploaded videos get the needed exposure to have those two questions answered. That initial exposure to get the needed impressions is not a level-playing field for all. The point is, a video getting millions of views is not necessarily synonymous with good quality information that transforms lives. Of course, there are popular videos with high quality health information too. But YouTube is

Google's platform, and they can do whatever they like with it. It's their call.

What I will say though, at the risk of self-praise, is that the views on my version of the nitric oxide dump routine are well justified. If anything, that video should do even better. There isn't a week that passes by that I don't get testimonials from all four corners of the globe, with tales of how that one video has helped one individual or another deal with their hypertension. The routine has helped thousands and thousands of people, and I am proud of it. I believe in nitric oxide, and I will do anything to promote its use for blood pressure control. It's free, so why wouldn't you imbibe it?

I am happy to be the champion of nitric oxide. In fact, my children should engrave "champion of nitric oxide" on my headstone when I depart this earth. That would make me very happy in the afterlife. Three folks got a Nobel Prize for the discovery of the molecule; why let it go to waste? So, promote its use I shall.

Here is something you should know about the nitric oxide dump exercises in order to get the maximum benefit from the routine: the routine does not make nitric oxide for you. What it does is it helps you to release nitric oxide from the stores into your bloodstream, in order for it to do what it is designed to do: relax the smooth muscle on the walls of your arteries, thereby lowering your blood pressure. What I am saying here is that you need to recruit *other* lifestyle measures into your daily routine that promote the production of that nitric oxide molecule in the first place, in order for the exercise to be effective. For instance, eating high-nitrate vegetables will move you in that direction.

Once your body has the nitric oxide stored up, the exercise routine simply unleashes it from the lining of your blood vessels, where it is stored, into the bloodstream. Once released into your bloodstream, it kicks into gear, doing its job of lowering your blood pressure.

So, what's this nitric oxide dump routine? If you are not familiar with the routine, simply go to YouTube and type "Nitric Oxide Dump Dr Joe" into the search box and it will pop up. The exercise is better watched than described – in fact, I encourage viewers to do the exercise with me in full flow.

The main attraction of the nitric oxide dump routine is that it is time efficient; it only takes four minutes to execute. You should be looking to do it three times a day, in the morning, afternoon and evening. Doing the routine three times a day totals twelve minutes. Can you sacrifice twelve minutes in a 24-hour day to look after your health? I'd like to think that's not too much to ask. While I said the routine is better seen than described, I will offer a brief description here. After all, this is a book, so you deserve the text version too.

There are four sub-routines to the nitric oxide dump exercise. Here they are:

1. The squat. Just regular squats. Remember to use the correct squatting technique. Very important. Do twenty reps.
2. Circular arm swing. Make a fist of your hands because the exercise requires your arms to be aerodynamic when you swing them in the air. You swing your two arms sideways above your head for the two fists to meet above your head. Then swing the arms back down in a circular manner for your two fists to meet in front of your body. Probably meeting just below or by your crotch. Repeat again. A complete circular swing is one rep. Do twenty reps.
3. Static forward march. Swing your arms forwards not together but alternately as though you are marching

forwards. Think soldiers marching forwards. But instead of marching forwards, you are standing still but swinging the arms forwards with your fist closed. When the right arm has swung forwards and returned followed by the left arm, that's one rep. Both arms must have swung forwards and back down meeting your thighs for a rep to be counted as one. Do twenty reps.

4. Shoulder press. Flex both arms at the elbow at shoulder level. Push both arms upwards together above your head to straighten them and lower them back down. Repeat again and again. Each upwards push and return to shoulder level is one rep. Do twenty reps.

You do the twenty reps of each of the sub-routines one after the other. In that order – squats, circular arm swing, static forward march, and shoulder press. Completion of the four sub-routines represents one set. Do three sets which would represent one nitric oxide dump exercise routine. You should do three sets in the morning, another three sets in the afternoon and one more three-set session in the evening.

Here is what you must do though. The nitric oxide dump routine is a high intensity interval training (HIIT) routine, but without the interval, meaning the speed is very important. The routine is usually completed in four minutes or less, and you should time yourself doing the routine. Anything more than four minutes suggests you are going too slow, meaning you need to increase the pace. Let me repeat this: speed is one reason why this routine works. Aim to finish each session within four minutes or less.

Please remember this: the nitric oxide dump routine, as simple as it is, shouldn't be underrated. It has helped thousands of people from all over the world, and it can help you too – simplicity works. Can you combine the nitric oxide dump routine with other exercises? Yes, you can, it's not a problem. Combine it with other aerobics, combine it with resistance training; it's all good. As for how long you can do this exercise for, put it this way: I've been doing this routine daily for the last four years at the time of writing, and I have no plans to give it up. Just keep going.

I'd like to say one last word about exercise for blood pressure reduction in general. There is no doubt that exercise, as a planned physical activity, reduces blood pressure in hypertensive individuals, and that the degree of reduction follows the law of initial values. Higher starting blood pressures obtain bigger reductions, and in fact, adults with hypertension can expect to have twice the blood pressure reductions experienced by prehypertensive individuals through exercise, and five times better blood pressure reductions compared with individuals with normal blood pressure[211]. That's the beauty of exercise.

Prescription

Exercise may seem like a curse word when you don't want to engage with it, but such an attitude would be ill-advised. If you have high blood pressure, you need exercise more than it needs you. Start small and gradually build it up; it can be fun when you get into your stride. Get yourself to a level on which you feel guilty for not exercising on your rest days, but you know your rest days are authorised. Once you start missing your exercise like a loved one on your rest days, you'll know you've hit the sweet spot.

Another way of knowing when you've hit the exercise happy spot is when you look out of your window to see a neighbour jogging past your property and feel jealous, wishing it was you. That's how I feel when driving to work; I see someone walking or running for their health, and I feel jealous, even though I have had my share of exercise that morning. You are always hungry for more when you hit the exercise dopamine spot. If, on the other hand, you are still finding it difficult to motivate yourself, use my nitric oxide dump exercise routine. It is the simplest exercise you can do, and the results you can get with such a simple routine are amazing, so long as you commit to doing it as I have prescribed.

Here is something that will sound like music to your ears: you do not have to commit to gym sessions if you don't want to. I don't do gyms personally. You can simply do home exercises and other outdoor exercises if weather permits.

All that I request of you is commit to fifteen- to twenty-minute exercise sessions twice a day, one session in the morning and another in the evening. If twice a day is too much to ask, simply do a thirty- to forty-minute session, either in the morning or the evening. Commit to doing one routine or a mix of routines six days a week, and rest on day seven to allow for recovery. That's all you need for blood pressure reduction purposes. Seriously, that's it.

> Question: When have you ever completed an exercise session and regretted it?
> Answer: Never!
> Just some food for thought!

CHAPTER 17

When Not To Check Your Blood Pressure

One of the highlights of the twentieth century was the invention that transformed the bulky sphygmomanometer to the portable blood pressure monitor. This invention made it possible for hypertensive individuals to own a device with which they could participate in their own blood pressure management. This was a welcome development, as patients having input into the management of their condition improves outcomes. Nice, but it does come with its own headache (not literally).

Here is what I mean: hypertensive individuals have arguably become *too* enthusiastic about their blood pressure monitoring, so much so that some individuals have been known to check their blood pressure up to twenty times a day. We have therefore progressed from the position of not checking blood pressure at all until a visit to the doctor's office to excessive checking, and neither position is good. They are extremes.

I made a video on this subject on YouTube and titled it "Stop Obsessing About Your Blood Pressure Number", because lately, it is an obsession, and such a degree of obsession is not healthy.

In the video, I suggested that individuals spend more of their energy dealing with the risk factors associated with hypertension rather than sitting idly and endlessly pushing the "start" button on their blood pressure monitor. The main outcome of this obsession is that it breeds anxiety, and the last thing you want when you are hypertensive is anxiety. Anxiety is not high blood pressure's friend at all, and once you've become anxious, your blood pressure readings will spin out of control. Remember those adrenaline and noradrenaline hormones, and let's not forget cortisol. These are stress hormones that won't do your blood pressure any favours.

Concentrate on getting better, rather than focusing on blood pressure numbers day in, day out. If you can sort out your risk factors, like your sedentary lifestyle, inflammatory diet, cholesterol, stress, smoking, diabetes, excess body fat etcetera, your blood pressure will fall in line. It's that simple, and then you won't have to stress over your blood pressure numbers any longer.

So, How Often To Check Your Blood Pressure?

Well, it depends on where you are in your healing journey. I liken blood pressure monitoring to a pilot managing a flight. When is the pilot most busy? At take-off and at landing. A pilot is usually very busy at take-off, but once the plane reaches the right altitude and the pilot is happy with everything, he can relax, take a bathroom break if needed. Not much happens when cruising at the right altitude; he occasionally glances at the controls to make sure all is good, but the next time he gets busy is when he is in preparation for landing and during the landing itself. The same applies to your blood pressure monitoring, except there is no landing. You simply cruise once your readings are under control.

At the start of your journey, you may need to check your blood pressure more often. Not as often as twenty times a day – that's just overkill – but maybe twice a day at a push to see whether there is a pattern of higher blood pressure at certain times of the day. This frequency should last no more than four to six weeks; once a pattern is established, move on to once a day. I usually suggest checking your blood pressure in the evenings before having your dinner because of the morning cortisol effect on your blood pressure, which artificially pushes up the readings. This is physiological, by the way, and from midday the cortisol effect will have worn off and your readings will no longer be physiologically influenced.

Another time you may want to check more often is when you introduce a new intervention, like a new exercise regime. Just like when your doctor adds a new medication to your current line-up, it makes sense to check to see how the new intervention is playing out. One more reason for frequent blood pressure checks is when you are putting data together for your next doctor's visit. Having a good amount of data spanning two to three weeks before your appointment gives your doctor something to work with, and if your doctor instructs you to gather lots more readings, then follow his/her instructions.

Also, when there is a stressful event in your life for instance bereavement, financial difficulties, relationship issues, new job, new house etcetera you may want to check about twice a day to see how the stress is impacting your blood pressure readings. Beyond these scenarios, it's hard to justify checking your blood pressure more than once a day.

Once you have your blood pressure under control, you should see yourself as someone at a cruising altitude, just like our pilot. At that point, checking two to three times a week is adequate. The point is, there is no need to obsess over your blood pressure readings. Keep your enthusiasm in check and keep anxiety at bay; do not allow hypertension to become your identity. You are worth more than that, and when you turn your blood pressure measurements into a habit, you are acquiring a new identity, and not an enviable one. You are you, and high blood pressure is just a small part of you – a small part that wants to shout out loud. Fortunately, you now have the tools to keep it quiet. So, curb your enthusiasm towards obsessive checking, and enthuse over a healthier lifestyle that will put a lid on your blood pressure concerns instead.

Now, to round off this penultimate chapter, I would like to talk about when *not* to check your blood pressure, because there are other factors at play when it comes to blood pressure readings. There are some factors that you have no control over, but the good news is that you have control over when to check your blood pressure and when not to. The circumstances I have mentioned below are guaranteed to give you high blood pressure readings, and are also guaranteed to upset you, so they are best avoided. These are physiological responses, and so the readings are temporary.

So, when should you not check your blood pressure? Here we go:

- Immediately after waking up from sleep. Arousal raises your blood pressure
- Soon after an exercise session – wait at least an hour before checking
- Soon after having a cigarette. You should be looking to quit smoking, by the way
- After having coffee or any other caffeinated beverage unless you are researching your response to caffeine
- Before, during and after watching any sporting event, especially when you are emotionally connected to one of the teams or participants

- When you are cold
- When you are hot
- After an argument, whether domestic or otherwise
- Following road rage
- After having a cold drink
- Soon after a shower or a bath (cold or hot)
- Soon after eating especially if it is a large meal
- Before making a presentation (public speaking) or soon after
- At work
- Whilst watching an emotionally charged TV show, documentary, or movie
- After reading an emotive piece in a novel, email, article or listening to an emotive podcast
- After listening to or watching a motivational speech
- After consuming alcohol
- When you are in pain regardless of the site

This list is not exhaustive. The point is that you want to be as relaxed as possible, devoid of any emotional encumbrances in order to have a reading that has no physiological interference. That's when you know your current blood pressure reading is one you can rely on to be accurate. I want you to feel confident when you are checking your blood pressure. Avoiding these awkward situations is one way of boosting your confidence.

Now let's wrap this up.

Closing Chapter

One thing you will have noticed in the course of reading this book is that there are several lifestyle intervention methods available to you if you are driven and have the motivation to lower your blood pressure. Choice is a good thing, but it can also be a problem too. Too many choices may result in overwhelm, leaving you wondering where to start.

My plan for you is to kick off your journey with three lifestyle measures and see how your blood pressure responds, and it doesn't hurt to start with the simplest.

Exercise is key to blood pressure reduction because hypertension loves an individual who is sedentary. So, one of the first measures to start off with will be an exercise routine. And if you are wondering what exercise to commence your journey with, well worry not because the nitric oxide dump exercise routine is here to help. The beauty of the nitric oxide dump is that it is time-efficient and very simple to do. The nitric oxide dump allows you to dip your toes into the exercise pool without fear of "drowning". Did I mention it only uses up four minutes of your precious time on each occasion?

The nitric oxide dump exercise routine is challenging but not overly demanding on your cardiovascular system. It makes a perfect starter exercise routine for lowering your blood pressure. Does it get the participant blood pressure reduction results? You bet it does. Therefore, that's one measure to put in your starter box. As you get more adept at the nitric oxide dump exercise routine, then it's time to add brisk walking. You may go back to the exercise chapter for the finer details but remember to target three miles per hour speed covering at least three miles on each occasion. If you want to take things to the next level with walking, then I suggest you get yourself a treadmill machine with an incline of at least twelve degrees and get walking on the treadmill five times a week. My recommended target treadmill speed will be three miles per hour and walk for forty-five minutes non-stop at an incline of fifteen degrees. But if your machine has a maximum incline of twelve degrees, then set it to that maximum incline. It's not enough but it will do if that's all you've got. The beauty of a treadmill acquisition is you stop worrying about the weather outside which may truncate your walking plans. You will never be a seasonal walker anymore once you get a treadmill for personal use. Again, even though I set you that target, you may not hit it at the beginning of your treadmill routine as a rookie walker. You may start off with a speed of one and half mile per hour speed with a more manageable incline of five degrees and that's okay too. After all you are just starting off, I wouldn't expect you to hit the lofty heights just yet. I never get tired of saying, start small and build up gradually.

What's next? How about herbal teas? Drinking tea is not a demanding task, is it? I don't think it is by my reckoning. So, incorporating drinking herbal teas, like hibiscus tea, rooibos tea, dandelion root tea and hawthorn tea for instance, into your daily lifestyle routine should be your next move. Look to consume at least three cups of each of those teas per day. The downside of using teas for blood pressure control is that the doses of the polyphenols from the teas can be small per drinking session. The way round that is to allow the teas to brew for a good while. A minimum of five minutes brewing time is desirable. Ideally longer brewing time is my recommendation. In fact, I let my tea bags remain in the cup till I drink the last drop from the cup. Using boiled water to make your herbal teas is unnegotiable, even if you like drinking your tea cold. Your starting point for tea preparation is boiled water. Could you combine different teas in one cup? Yes, you can, and I encourage that practice all day long.

The third simplest lifestyle measure will be to add one of the juices for high blood pressure reduction measures into the plan. Either you start juicing your beetroot or you juice your celery. It doesn't have to be one or the other by the way. You can alternate the juices. Have celery juice today and beetroot juice the day after. This is also simple to adopt and gets you off to a flying start. Remember the recommended doses of the juices – 8 oz (250 ml) for beetroot juice and 16 oz (500 ml) for the celery juice. If you don't have a juicer, invest in one and in particular one that is easy to clean after use, so you don't get exasperated washing it up after each use. I want you to have fun doing this rather than see it as a chore.

Start off with those three measures above and for some of you, they may be all you need to see the results you are after. The journey doesn't end there though. Some people will need more and that's where your diet will need an overhaul – probably a complete overhaul. Go back to the diet chapter and pick on just three ideas to start off with, so you don't suffer from overwhelm. Whilst you are ruminating over that, how about you have the green smoothies at midday every day. Use them as a meal replacement or as the main part of your lunch. Now you are beginning to see how easy it is to incorporate these changes into your lifestyle.

And, of course, your sleep needs fixing too if you have sleep problems. By that I am referring to those with difficulties falling asleep or staying asleep for a reasonable number of hours throughout the night. Sleep is all about quantity and quality. Both sleep quantity and quality matter – you need both for good blood pressure management.

One reason you want to fix your sleep issues is that it does impact your stress management. Poor sleep leads to poor stress management, in particular anxiety control. We are aiming to let our parasympathetic nervous system dominate our sympathetic nervous system for better blood pressure control. Managing your sleep and your stress effectively is imperative and you must not ignore it. I am not saying it is an easy thing to do but putting into place the various techniques and steps I talked about in the relevant chapters will get you there. It may be an on-going project, but you will arrive at your destination with practice.

Of course, the "don'ts" are just as important as the "dos" when it comes to blood pressure reduction. So, avoiding caffeinated beverages, supplements with xenadrine, ephedrine, bitter orange etc. and cutting out sugar and processed foods are just as important as investing forty minutes a day engaging in some form of exercise or at the very least doing the nitric oxide dump exercise three times a day which will total twelve minutes. It's about adopting a cohesive approach.

One more thing I really need to point out. In the book, I mentioned a lot of studies related to blood pressure control. I also outlined the reductions in both systolic and diastolic blood pressure research findings. You will have noticed some interventions for instance producing an eight-point drop in systolic blood pressure readings and maybe a three-point drop in diastolic readings. To some people that might not look impressive enough as they may be looking for a twenty-point drop in systolic readings as an impressive number.

Here is what you should know regarding blood pressure reductions with lifestyle modification. We aim for an additive effect with a lifestyle approach to blood pressure management. We are looking to have a couple of measures help each other out to get us to the finish line. If one measure gets us there, then that's great. For instance, I have people who have used just the nitric oxide dump exercise routine to do the job. Fantastic!

But for a lot of hypertensive individuals, they will need more than one lifestyle measure to get the result they need. Each lifestyle measure brings a modest contribution to the plate, and you will end up with a cumulative final blood pressure reduction figure that will impress both you and your doctor. So, whereas an eight-point reduction in systolic may not sound like much, but that could mean dropping your systolic reading from 157 mmHg to 149 mmHg in real terms. Add another life-style measure that does something similar, and you suddenly see a reduction of your systolic to 141 mmHg. The principle here is about little victories adding up to a bigger victory.

So, it is best not to have a greedy mindset and be one of those looking for the only intervention that will give us one big victory. If we have an attitude like that, we set ourselves up for disappointment if we don't get that eye popping triumph we were expecting. That will be the wrong mindset. This is one process where you should think small and maybe an intervention will over-deliver but if it delivers small results, we don't feel discouraged because that's what we anticipated.

Here is something else I want you to take home. You want to avoid the concept of tunnel vision. What do I mean by that? A tunnel vision approach is one that is hopelessly focused on blood pressure reduction alone. Practically every lifestyle measure in this book has effects beyond blood pressure and even beyond your entire cardiovascular system. The interventions on offer here positively affect your brain health, your liver health, your kidney health, the health of your pancreas, your gut health etc. The benefits of these lifestyle measures are far reaching meaning your overall health will be touched in a positive way by all of these interventions. You may be bringing down those blood pressure numbers by working really hard, but your brain will also be singing halleluiah for giving it the nourishment it's been lacking for decades which may just reduce your risk of Alzheimer's disease when you get older. And your liver will be ridding itself of that accumulated fat that's preventing it from performing its metabolic functions effectively. Your gut microbiome will be thanking you for feeding them with all the fiber they need. Hence you should have a broader outlook for what we are trying to achieve here and that should spur you on which brings me to another piece of advice.

And that is the message of consistency. Lowering your blood pressure naturally is a marathon; it's not a sprint. To get results you have to stay consistent in your pursuit of results. You have to dedicate yourself to the course. A half-hearted approach will lead to poor results, but a robust attitude will yield those blood pressure numbers that we all yearn for. Being consistent for two weeks and slacking off for the next one month is an example of a half-hearted approach. Asking yourself a simple question like, "is this good for my blood pressure?" in everything you do is a nice way to stay on track and be consistent in your application. I will go as far as labelling our new way of life as a "better blood pressure" lifestyle because it is a lifestyle after all, and this lifestyle is for life, not just for the month of January.

Well done for completing this book. I thank you for your custom, but reading a book is one thing and doing is another. I do not want you to fall into the trap of procrastination; the hard work begins now, and the sooner you start, the better.

Having read this book, your knowledge of blood pressure and natural blood pressure management is way better than the man next door. You now have the tools in this book to conquer blood pressure and reverse it. It's a journey, and it may not be smooth, but sticking to the plan will see you through.

Even though your sojourn through this book is over, I won't just leave you hanging. I have set up a communication tool for my customers. It's an email list where we can stay in touch with each other.

I encourage you to join it. Through that communication tool, you will be the first to know when the second book that complements this very book you have just read gets published. The second book will be the *90-day Blueprint to Lowering Your Blood Pressure* and it shall provide you with a weekly roadmap that will ease the way for your progress. And, of course, be the first to know when subsequent editions of this book are published too. Also, if you bought the digital edition of this book, you may want to know when to grab the hard copy. I will let you know where to go to get your copy easily without fuss. All of that information will be communicated to you via email as well as when I have anything interesting to say. So, do join this communication superhighway please. Thank you very much.

How do you do that? Well, go to:

https://drjoeconnect.com

Please go there to sign up now before you forget. Talk to you over there.

Disclaimer:

Information in this book is provided for informational and educational purposes only. This information is not intended as a substitute for the advice provided by your physician or other healthcare professional or any information contained on or in any product mentioned or recommended in the book. Do not use the information in the book for diagnosing or treating a health problem or disease, or prescribing medication or other treatment. Always speak with your physician or other healthcare professional before taking any advice or nutritional or herbal supplement, or using any treatment suggested or recommended in this book. If you have or suspect that you have a medical problem, contact your health care provider promptly. Do not disregard professional medical advice or delay in seeking professional advice because of something you have read in this book. Information provided in this book and the use of any products or services mentioned or recommended in this book does not create a doctor-patient relationship between you and Dr Joseph Amagada or the publishers. Information and statements regarding dietary supplements have not been evaluated by the Food and Drug Administration and are not intended to diagnose, treat, cure, or prevent any disease

All information provided in this book has been provided in good faith. We make no representation or warranty of any kind, expressed, or implied regarding the accuracy, reliability, adequacy, validity, or completeness of all the information provided in this book. Under no circumstances shall we or the publishers have any liability to you for any loss or damage of any kind as a result of consuming and applying the information in this book. Your use and application of the contents of this book is purely at your own risk.

References

1. More than 700 million people with untreated hypertension [Internet]. www.who.int. 2021. https://www.who.int/news/item/25-08-2021-more-than-700-million-people-with-untreated-hypertension

2. Hypertension prevalence estimates in England, 2017 [Internet]. 2017. https://assets.publishing.service.gov.uk/government/uploads/system/uploads/attachment_data/file/873605/Summary_of_hypertension_prevalence_estimates_in_England__1_.pdf

3. High Blood Pressure Facts [Internet]. Centers for Disease Control and Prevention. 2021. https://www.cdc.gov/bloodpressure/facts.htm

4. Underlying Cause of Death, 1999–2020 [Internet]. CDC WONDER Online Database. Centers for Disease Control and Prevention; 2020. http://wonder.cdc.gov/ucd-icd10.html

4a. Hay J. A British Medical Association Lecture on THE SIGNIFICANCE OF A RAISED BLOOD PRESSURE. BMJ. 1931. pp 43–47

4b. Moser M. Historical Perspectives on the Management of Hypertension. The Journal of Clinical Hypertension [Internet]. 2006. https://onlinelibrary.wiley.com/doi/epdf/10.1111/j.1524-6175.2006.05836.x

5. Lemley MA. The Myth of the Sole Inventor [Internet]. SSRN. 2011. https://papers.ssrn.com/sol3/papers.cfm?abstract_id=1856610

6. Thompson D. Forget Edison: This is How History's Greatest Inventions Really Happened [Internet]. The Atlantic. 2012. https://www.theatlantic.com/business/archive/2012/06/

forget-edison-this-is-how-historys-greatest-inventions-really-happened/258525/

7. Haddad K. Stories behind some of most important, useful inventions in human history [Internet]. WDIV. 2019. https://www.clickondetroit.com/lifestyle/2019/07/16/stories-behind-some-of-most-important-useful-inventions-in-human-history/

8. William Harvey [Internet]. Wikipedia. 2020. https://en.wikipedia.org/wiki/William_Harvey

9. Stephen Hales [Internet]. Wikipedia. 2020. https://en.wikipedia.org/wiki/Stephen_Hales

10. Lewis O. Stephen Hales and the measurement of blood pressure. The Journal of Human Hypertension. 1994; 8(12) pp 865–871

11. Smith IB. The impact of Stephen Hales on medicine. J R Soc Med. 1993; 86(6) pp 349–352

12. Scipione Riva-Rocci [Internet]. Wikipedia. 2020. https://en.wikipedia.org/wiki/Scipione_Riva-Rocci

13. Nikolai Korotkov [Internet]. Wikipedia. 2020. https://en.wikipedia.org/wiki/Nikolai_Korotkov

14. Esunge PM. From blood pressure to hypertension: the history of research. J R Soc Med. 1991; 84(10) pp 621

15. Charles L, Triscott J, Dobbs B. Secondary Hypertension: Discovering the Underlying Cause. Am Fam Physician. 2017; 96(7) pp 453–461

16. Cushing's Syndrome [Internet]. Your Hormones https://www.yourhormones.info/endocrine-conditions/cushing-s-syndrome/

17. Phaeochromocytoma [Internet]. Your Hormones https://www.yourhormones.info/endocrine-conditions/phaeochromocytoma/

18. Aldosterone [Internet]. Your Hormones https://www.yourhormones.info/hormones/aldosterone/

19. Tarray R, Saleem S, Yousuf I, Gulnar A, Laway B, Verma S. Role of insulin resistance in essential hypertension. Cardiovascular Endocrinology & Metabolism. 2014; 3(4) pp 129–133

20. Wang F, Han L, Hu D. Fasting insulin, insulin resistance and risk of hypertension in the general population: A meta-analysis. Clinica Chimica Acta. 2017; 464 pp 57–63

21. Bamaiyi AJ, Woodiwiss AJ, Peterson V, Gomes M, Libhaber CD, Sareli P, Norton GR. Insulin resistance influences the impact

of hypertension on left ventricular diastolic dysfunction in a community sample. Clinical Cardiology. 2019; 42(2) pp 305–311

22. Chobanian AV, Bakris GL, Black HR, Cushman WC, Green LA, Izzo Jr JL, Jones DW, Materson BJ, Oparil S, Wright Jr JT, Roccella EJ. Seventh Report of the Joint National Committee on Prevention, Detection, Evaluation, and Treatment of High Blood Pressure. Hypertension. 2003; 42(6) pp 1206–1252

23. Johnson AG. NSAIDs and Increased Blood Pressure. Drug Safety. 1997; 17(5) pp 277–289

24. Whelton A. Nephrotoxicity of nonsteroidal anti-inflammatory drugs: physiologic foundations and clinical implications. The American Journal of Medicine. 1999; 106(5) pp 13S–24S

25. Linde K, Ramirez G, Mulrow CD, Pauls A, Weidenhammer W, Melchart D. St John's wort for depression—an overview and meta-analysis of randomised clinical trials. BMJ. 1996; 313(7052) pp 253–258

26. Butterweck V. Mechanism of Action of St John's Wort in Depression. CNS Drugs. 2003; 17(8) pp 539–562

27. Patel S, Robinson R, Burk M. Hypertensive crisis associated with St. John's Wort. The American Journal of Medicine. 2002: 112(6) pp 507–508

28. Allcock E, Cowdery J. Hypertension induced by liquorice tea. Case Reports. 2015: bcr2015209926

29. Penninkilampi R, Eslick EM, Eslick, GD. The association between consistent licorice ingestion, hypertension and hypo-kalaemia: a systematic review and meta-analysis. The Journal of Human Hypertension. 2017; 31(11) pp 699–707

30. Can eating too much liquorice be bad for you? [Internet]. NHS. 2018. https://www.nhs.uk/common-health-questions/food-and-diet/can-eating-too-much-black-liquorice-be-bad-for-you/

31. Bitter Orange [Internet]. NCCIH. https://www.nccih.nih.gov/health/bitter-orange

32. Bui LT, Nguyen DT, Ambrose PJ. Blood Pressure and Heart Rate Effects Following a Single Dose of Bitter Orange. Annals of Pharmacotherapy. 2006; 40(1) pp 53–57

33. Gange CA, Madias C, Felix-Getzik EM, Weintraub AR, Estes NAM. Variant Angina Associated With Bitter Orange in a

Dietary Supplement. [Internet]. Mayo Clinic Proceedings. 2006. https://www.mayoclinicproceedings.org/article/S0025-6196(11)61904-6/fulltext

34. https://core.ac.uk/download/pdf/195070715.pdf

35. Gadde KM. Current pharmacotherapy for obesity: extrapolation of clinical trials data to practice. Expert Opinion on Pharmacotherapy. 2014; 15(6) pp 809–822

36. Jensen MD, Ryan DH, Apovian CM, Ard JD, Comuzzie AG, Donato KA, Hu FB, Hubbard VS, Jakicic JM, Kushner RF, Loria CM. 2013 AHA/ACC/TOS Guideline for the Management of Overweight and Obesity in Adults: A Report of the American College of Cardiology/American Heart Association Task Force on Practice Guidelines and The Obesity Society. Journal of the American College of Cardiology. 2014; 63(25) pp 2985–3023

37. Gadde KM, Martin CK, Berthoud HR, Heymsfield SB. Obesity: Pathophysiology and Management. Journal of the American College of Cardiology. 2018; 71(1) pp 69–84

38. Kim KK, Cho HG, Kang HC, Youn BB, Lee KR. Effects on weight reduction and safety of short-term phentermine administration in Korean obese people. Yonsei Medical Journal. 2006; 47(5) pp 614–625

39. Kang JG, Park CY, Kang JH, Park YW, Park SW. Randomized controlled trial to investigate the effects of a newly developed formulation of phentermine diffuse-controlled release for obesity. Diabetes, Obesity and Metabolism. 2010; 12(10) pp 876–882

40. Aronne LJ, Wadden TA, Peterson C, Winslow D, Odeh S, Gadde KM. Evaluation of phentermine and topiramate versus phentermine/topiramate extended-release in obese adults. Obesity. 2013; 21(11) pp 2163–2171

41. Cohen JB, Gadde KM. Weight loss medications in the treatment of obesity and hypertension. Current Hypertension Reports. 2019; 21(2) pp 11906–11919

42. Hollander-Rodriguez JC, Montjoy HL, Smedra B, Prouty JP, Hamilton A, Guthmann R. Do oral decongestants have a clinically significant effect on BP in patients with hypertension? Journal of Family Practice. 2017; 66(6) E1–E2

43. Chua SS, Benrimoj SI. Non-prescription sympathomimetic agents and hypertension. Medical Toxicology and Adverse Drug Experiment 1988; 3(5) pp 387–417

44. Cantu C, Arauz A, Murillo-Bonilla LM, López M, Barinagarrementeria F. Stroke associated with sympathomimetics contained in over-the-counter cough and cold drugs. Stroke. 2003; 34(7) pp 1667–1672

45. Bradley JG. Nonprescription drugs and hypertension. Which ones affect blood pressure? Postgraduate Medicine. 1991; 89(6) pp 195–197

46. Walker S. New Medications in the Treatment of Acute Migraine. Hospital Pharmacy. 2019; 54(4) pp 229–231

47. Charles AC, Baca SM. Cortical spreading depression and migraine. Nature Reviews Neurololgy. 2013; 9(11) pp 637–644

48. Geppetti P, Rossi E, Chiarugi A, Benemei S. Antidromic vasodilatation and the migraine mechanism. The Journal of Headache and Pain. 2012; 13(2) pp 103–111

49. Kuo CY, Yen MF, Chen LS, Fann CY, Chiu YH, Chen HH, Pan SL. Increased risk of hemorrhagic stroke in patients with migraine: a population-based cohort study. PLoS One. 2013; 8(1) pp 552–553

50. Gilmore B, Michael M. Treatment of acute migraine headache. American Family Physician. 2011; 83(3) pp 271–280

51. Rudorfer MV. Monoamine oxidase inhibitors: reversible and irreversible. Psychopharmacol Bull. 1992; 28(1) pp 45–57

52. Outfitters CM, Rockville M, BioPharma C, Corcept Therapeutics G, Lundbeck M, Organon P. Revisiting monoamine oxidase inhibitors. J Clin Psychiatry. 2007; 68(8) pp 35–41

53. Fiori MG. Tricyclic antidepressants: a review of their toxicology. Current Developments in Psychopharmacology. 1977; 4 pp 71–110

54. Buoli M, Serati M, Cahn W. Alternative pharmacological strategies for adult ADHD treatment: a systematic review. Expert Review of Neurotherapeutics. 2016; 16(2) pp 131–144

55. Ritchie H, Roser M, Dattani S. Mental health [Internet]. Our World in Data. 2018. https://ourworldindata.org/mental-health

56. Crookes DM, Demmer RT, Keyes KM, Koenen KC, Suglia SF. Depressive Symptoms, Antidepressant Use, and Hypertension in Young Adulthood. Epidemiology. 2018; 29(4) pp 547–555

57. Alomar M, Palaian S, Al-Tabakha MM. Pharmacovigilance in perspective: drug withdrawals, data mining and policy implications. F1000Research. 2019; 8

58. Quigley EM. Cisapride: what can we learn from the rise and fall of a prokinetic? Journal of Digestive Diseases. 2011; 12(3) pp 147–156

59. Humbert X, Fedrizzi S, Chrétien B, Sassier M, Bagheri H, Combret S, Drici MD, Le Bas F, Puddu PE, Alexandre J. Hypertension induced by serotonin reuptake inhibitors: analysis of two pharmacovigilance databases. Fundamental & Clinical Pharmacology. 2019; 33(3) pp 296–302

60. Oparil S. Hypertension and oral contraceptives. The Journal of Cardiovascular Medicine. 1981; 6(4) pp 384–387

61. Woods JW. Oral contraceptives and hypertension. Hypertension. 1988; 11(3 Pt 2) pp 11-15.

62. White K, Potter JE, Hopkins K, Amastae J, Grossman D. Hypertension among oral contraceptive users in El Paso, Texas. Journal of Health Care for the Poor and Underserved. 2013; 24(4) pp 1511–1521

63. Lim KG, Isles CG, Hodsman GP, Lever AF, Robertson JW. Malignant hypertension in women of childbearing age and its relation to the contraceptive pill. *Br Med J (Clin Res Ed). 1987;* 294(6579) pp 1057–1059

64. Grossman D, Fernandez L, Hopkins K, Amastae J, Garcia SG, Potter JE. Accuracy of self-screening for contraindications to combined oral contraceptive use. Obstetrics and Gynecology. 2008; 112(3) pp 572–578

65. Gilbert RM. Caffeine consumption. Progress in clinical and biological research. 1984; 158 pp 185–213

66. List of countries by coffee production [Internet]. Wikipedia. 2020 https://en.wikipedia.org/wiki/List_of_countries_by_coffee_production

67. The history of coffee [Internet]. National Coffee Association of U.S.A., Inc. 2020 https://www.ncausa.org/about-coffee/history-of-coffee

68. History of coffee [Internet]. Wikipedia. 2020 https://en.wikipedia.org/wiki/History_of_coffee

69. Boston Tea Party [Internet]. Wikipedia. 2020 https://en.wikipedia.org/wiki/Boston_Tea_Party

70. Nicoli MC, Anese M, Manzocco L, Lerici CR. Antioxidant properties of coffee brews in relation to the roasting degree. LWT-Food Science and Technology. 1997; 30(3) pp 292–297

71. Yashin A, Yashin Y, Wang JY, Nemzer B. Antioxidant and Antiradical Activity of Coffee. Antioxidants. 2013; 2(4) pp 230–245

72. Rodríguez-Artalejo F, López-García E. Coffee Consumption and Cardiovascular Disease: A Condensed Review of Epidemiological Evidence and Mechanisms. Journal of Agricultural and Food Chemistry. 2018; 66(21) pp 5257–5263

73. Zhou A, Hyppönen E. Long-term coffee consumption, caffeine metabolism genetics, and risk of cardiovascular disease: a prospective analysis of up to 347,077 individuals and 8368 cases. The American Journal of Clinical Nutrition. 2019; 109(3) pp 509–516

74. Cornelis MC, El-Sohemy A, Kabagambe EK, Campos H. Coffee, CYP1A2 genotype, and risk of myocardial infarction. JAMA. 2006; 295(10) pp 1135–1141

75. Mesas AE, Leon-Muñoz LM, Rodriguez-Artalejo F, Lopez-Garcia E. The effect of coffee on blood pressure and cardiovascular disease in hypertensive individuals: a systematic review and meta-analysis. The American Journal of Clinical Nutrition. 2011; 94(4) pp 1113–1126

76. Jeong DU, Dimsdale JE. The effects of caffeine on blood pressure in the work environment. American Journal of Hypertension. 1990; 3(10 Pt 1) pp 749–753

77. Pincomb GA, Lovallo WR, Passey RB, Wilson MF. Effect of behavior state on caffeine's ability to alter blood pressure. The American Journal of Cardiology. 1988; 61(10) pp 798–802

78. Hartley TR, Sung BH, Pincomb GA, Whitsett TL, Wilson MF, Lovallo WR. Hypertension risk status and effect caffeine on blood pressure. Hypertension. 2000; 36(1) pp 137–141

79. Joint National Committee on Prevention, Detection, Evaluation, and Treatment of High Blood Pressure. The 6th Report of the Joint National Committee on Prevention, Detection, Evaluation, and Treatment of High Blood Pressure. Arch Intern Med. 1997; 157 pp 2413–2446

80. Lovallo WR, Al'Absi M, Blick K, Whitsett TL, Wilson MF. Stress-like adrenocorticotropin responses to caffeine in young healthy men. Pharmacology Biochemistry and Behavior. 1996; 55(3) pp 365–369

81. Lovallo WR, Whitsett TL, Al'Absi M, Sung BH, Vincent AS, Wilson MF. Caffeine stimulation of cortisol secretion across the waking hours in relation to caffeine intake levels. Psychosomatic Medicine. 2005; 67(5) pp 734–739

82. Lovallo WR, Farag NH, Vincent AS, Thomas TL, Wilson MF. Cortisol responses to mental stress, exercise, and meals following caffeine intake in men and women. Pharmacology Biochemistry and Behavior. 2006; 83(3) pp 441–447

83. Van Soeren M, Mohr T, Kjaer M, Graham TE. Acute effects of caffeine ingestion at rest in humans with impaired epinephrine responses. Journal of Applied Physiology. 1996; 80(3) pp 999–1005

84. Joint National Committee on Prevention, Detection, Evaluation, and Treatment of High Blood Pressure. The Seventh Report of the Joint National Committee on Prevention, Detection, Evaluation, and Treatment of High Blood Pressure: the JNC 7 report. JAMA. 2003; 289 pp 2560–2572

85. 2017 ACC/AHA/AAPA/ABC/ACPM/AGS/APhA/ASH/ASPC/NMA/PCNA Guideline for the Prevention, Detection, Evaluation, and Management of High Blood Pressure in Adults: Executive Summary: A Report of the American College of Cardiology/American Heart Association Task Force on Clinical Practice Guidelines. Journal of the American College of Cardiology. 2018; 71 pp 2199–2269

86. Whelton PK, Carey RM, Aronow WS, Casey DE, Collins KJ, Himmelfarb C. 2017 ACC/AHA/AAPA/ABC/ACPM/AGS/APhA/ASH/ASPC/NMA/PCNA Guideline for the Prevention, Detection, Evaluation, and Management of High Blood Pressure in Adults: Executive Summary: A Report of the American College of Cardiology/American Heart Association Task Force on Clinical Practice Guidelines. Hypertension. 2018; 71(6) pp 1269–1324

87. Pereira da Silva H, Bonilha A, Barretti P, Silva R, Burgugi V, dos Santos V, Cuadrado L. White-coat and masked hypertension

diagnoses in chronic kidney disease patients. The Journal of Clinical Hypertension. 2020; 22(7) pp 1202–1207

88. The North Star: Polaris [Internet]. Space. 2017 https://www.space.com/15567-north-star-polaris.html

89. Hermida RC, Ayala DE, Smolensky MH, Fernández JR, Mojón A, Portaluppi F. Chronotherapy with conventional blood pressure medications improves management of hypertension and reduces cardiovascular and stroke risks. Hypertension Research. 2016; 39(5) pp 277–292

90. Fagard RH, Thijs L, Staessen JA, Clement DL, De Buyzere ML, De Bacquer DA. Prognostic significance of ambulatory blood pressure in hypertensive patients with history of cardiovascular disease. Blood Pressure Monitoring. 2008; 13(6) pp 325–332

91. Pai AU, Chakrapani M, Bhaskaran U, Kamath P. Study of home-monitored night blood pressure and its correlation with left ventricular hypertrophy in treatment-naive hypertensive patients. Singapore Medical Journal. 2012; 53(2) pp 95–98

92. Renin release [Internet]. Science Direct. https://www.science-direct.com/topics/medicine-and-dentistry/renin-release

93. Angiotensin [Internet]. Your Hormones. 2016 https://www.yourhormones.info/hormones/angiotensin/

94. Lackland DT. Racial differences in hypertension: implications for high blood pressure management. The American Journal of the Medical Sciences. 2014; 348(2) pp 135–138

95. The Declaration of Independence, 1776 [Internet]. Office of the Historian. 2018 https://history.state.gov/milestones/1776-1783/declaration

96. DASH Eating Plan [Internet]. NHLBI. 2019 https://www.nhlbi.nih.gov/health-topics/dash-eating-plan

97. Appel LJ, Moore TJ, Obarzanek E, Vollmer WM, Svetkey LP, Sacks FM, Bray GA, Vogt TM, Cutler JA, Windhauser MM, Lin PH. A clinical trial of the effects of dietary patterns on blood pressure. New England Journal of Medicine. 1997; 336(16) pp 1117–1124

98. Appel LJ, Champagne CM, Harsha DW, Cooper LS, Obarzanek E, Elmer PJ, Stevens VJ, Vollmer WM, Lin PH, Svetkey LP, Young DR. Effects of comprehensive lifestyle modification on

blood pressure control: main results of the PREMIER clinical trial. JAMA. 2003; 289 pp 2083–2093

99. Ketogenic diet [Internet]. Wikipedia. 2020 https://en.wikipedia.org/wiki/Ketogenic_diet

100. Martin-McGill KJ, Bresnahan R, Levy RG, Cooper PN. Ketogenic diets for drug-resistant epilepsy. Cochrane Database of Systematic Reviews. 2020; Art. No.: CD001903

101. Bueno NB, de Melo IS, de Oliveira SL, da Rocha Ataide T. Very-low-carbohydrate ketogenic diet v. low-fat diet for long-term weight loss: a meta-analysis of randomised controlled trials. British Journal of Nutrition. 2013; 110(7) pp 1178–1187

102. Westerterp-Plantenga MS, Nieuwenhuizen A, Tome D, Soenen S, Westerterp KR. Dietary protein, weight loss, and weight maintenance. Annual Review of Nutrition. 2009; 29 pp 21–41

103. Veldhorst M, Smeets AJ, Soenen S, Hochstenbach-Waelen A, Hursel R, Diepvens K, Lejeune M, Luscombe-Marsh N, Westerterp-Plantenga M. Protein-induced satiety: effects and mechanisms of different proteins. Physiology & Behavior. 2008; 94(2) pp 300–307

104. Sumithran P, Prendergast LA, Delbridge E, Purcell K, Shulkes A, Kriketos A, Proietto J. Ketosis and appetite-mediating nutrients and hormones after weight loss. European Journal of Clinical Nutrition. 2013; 67(7) pp 759–764

105. Johnstone AM, Horgan GW, Murison SD, Bremner DM, Lobley GE. Effects of a high-protein ketogenic diet on hunger, appetite, and weight loss in obese men feeding ad libitum. The American Journal of Clinical Nutrition. 2008; 87(1) pp 44–55

106. Veldhorst MA, Westerterp-Plantenga MS, Westerterp KR. Gluconeogenesis and energy expenditure after a high-protein, carbohydrate-free diet. The American Journal of Clinical Nutrition. 2009; 90(3) pp 519–526

107. Cahill Jr GF. Fuel metabolism in starvation. Annual Review of Nutrition. 2006; 26 pp 1–22

108. Feinman RD, Fine EJ. Nonequilibrium thermodynamics and energy efficiency in weight loss diets. Theoretical Biology and Medical Modelling. 2007; 4(1) pp 1–3

109. Wing RR, Hill JO. Successful weight loss maintenance. Annual Review of Nutrition. 2001; 21(1) pp 323–341

110. Paoli A, Bianco A, Grimaldi KA, Lodi A, Bosco G. Long term successful weight loss with a combination biphasic ketogenic Mediterranean diet and Mediterranean diet maintenance protocol. Nutrients. 2013; 5(12) pp 5205–5217

111. Pandit R, Beerens S, Adan RA. Role of leptin in energy expenditure: the hypothalamic perspective. American Journal of Physiology-Regulatory, Integrative and Comparative Physiology. 2017; 312(6) pp R938–R947

112. Jenkins AB, Markovic TP, Fleury A, Campbell LV. Carbohydrate intake and short-term regulation of leptin in humans. Diabetologia. 1997; 40(3) pp 348–351

113. Dirlewanger M, di Vetta V, Guenat E, Battilana P, Seematter G, Schneiter P, Jéquier E, Tappy L. Effects of short-term carbohydrate or fat overfeeding on energy expenditure and plasma leptin concentrations in healthy female subjects. International Journal of Obesity. 2000; 24(11) pp 1413–1418

114. Thompson RC, Allam AH, Lombardi GP, Wann LS, Sutherland ML, Sutherland JD, Soliman MA, Frohlich B, Mininberg DT, Monge JM, Vallodolid CM. Atherosclerosis across 4000 years of human history: the Horus study of four ancient populations. The Lancet. 2013; 381(9873) pp 1211–1222

115. Jönsson T, Granfeldt Y, Ahrén B, Branell UC, Pålsson G, Hansson A, Söderström M, Lindeberg S. Beneficial effects of a Paleolithic diet on cardiovascular risk factors in type 2 diabetes: a randomized cross-over pilot study. Cardiovascular Diabetology. 2009; 8(1) pp 1–4

116. Watanabe F, Katsura H, Takenaka S, Fujita T, Abe K, Tamura Y, Nakatsuka T, Nakano Y. Pseudovitamin B12 is the predominant cobamide of an algal health food, spirulina tablets. Journal of Agricultural and Food Chemistry. 1999; 47(11) pp 4736–4741

117. Watanabe F. Vitamin B12 sources and bioavailability. Experimental Biology and Medicine. 2007; 232(10) pp 1266–1274

118. Li D. Effect of the vegetarian diet on non-communicable diseases. Journal of the Science of Food and Agriculture. 2014; 94(2) pp 169–173

119. Brenna JT. Efficiency of conversion of alpha-linolenic acid to long chain n-3 fatty acids in man. Current Opinion in Clinical Nutrition & Metabolic Care. 2002; 5(2) pp 127–132

120. Gerster H. Can adults adequately convert alpha-linolenic acid (18:3n-3) to eicosapentaenoic acid (20:5n-3) and docosahexaenoic acid (22:6n-3)? International Journal for Vitamin and Nutrition Research. 1998; 68(3) pp 159–173

121. Burdge GC. Metabolism of alpha-linolenic acid in humans. Prostaglandins, Leukotrienes and Essential Fatty Acids. 2006; 75(3) pp 161–168

122. Miller PE, Van Elswyk M, Alexander DD. Long-Chain Omega-3 Fatty Acids Eicosapentaenoic Acid and Docosahexaenoic Acid and Blood Pressure: A Meta-Analysis of Randomized Controlled Trials. American Journal of Hypertension. 2014; 27(7) pp 885–896

123. Jain AP, Aggarwal KK, Zhang PY. Omega-3 fatty acids and cardiovascular disease. European Review for Medical and Pharmacological Sciences. 2015; 19(3) pp 441–445

124. Najjar RS, Moore CE, Montgomery BD. A defined, plant-based diet utilized in an outpatient cardiovascular clinic effectively treats hypercholesterolemia and hypertension and reduces medications. Clinical Cardiology. 2018; 41(3) pp 307–313

125. Report of the Dietary Guidelines Advisory Committee on the Dietary Guidelines for Americans, 2010. U.S. Department of Agriculture, Agricultural Research Service. 2011

126. Fulgoni III VL, Keast DR, Bailey RL, Dwyer J. Foods, fortificants, and supplements: Where do Americans get their nutrients? The Journal of Nutrition. 2011; 141(10) pp 1847–1854

127. Staruschenko A. Beneficial Effects of High Potassium: Contribution of Renal Basolateral K+ Channels. Hypertension. 2018; 71(6) pp 1015–1022

128. Addison WL. The Use of Sodium Chloride, Potassium Chloride, Sodium Bromide, and Potassium Bromide in Cases of Arterial Hypertension which are Amenable to Potassium Chloride. Canadian Medical Association Journal. 1928; 18(3) pp 281–285

129. Houston MC. The importance of potassium in managing hypertension. Current Hypertension Reports. 2011; 13(4) pp 309–317

130. Dickinson HO, Nicolson DJ, Campbell F, Beyer FR, Mason J. Potassium supplementation for the management of primary hypertension in adults. Cochrane Database of Systematic Reviews. 2006; 19(3) CD004641

131. Touyz RM. Role of magnesium in the pathogenesis of hypertension. Molecular Aspects of Medicine. 2003; 24(1–3) pp 107–136

132. Houston M. The role of magnesium in hypertension and cardiovascular disease. The Journal of Clinical Hypertension. 2011; 13(11) pp 843–847

133. Patki PS, Singh J, Gokhale SV, Bulakh PM, Shrotri DS, Patwardhan B. Efficacy of potassium and magnesium in essential hypertension: a double-blind, placebo controlled, crossover study. BMJ. 1990; 301(6751) pp 521–523

134. Hatzistavri LS, Sarafidis PA, Georgianos PI, Tziolas IM, Aroditis CP, Zebekakis PE, Pikilidou MI, Lasaridis AN. Oral magnesium supplementation reduces ambulatory blood pressure in patients with mild hypertension. American Journal of Hypertension. 2001; 22(10) pp 1070–1075

135. Qu XM, Wu ZF, Pang BX, Jin LY, Qin LZ, Wang SL. From Nitrate to Nitric Oxide: The Role of Salivary Glands and Oral Bacteria. Journal of Dental Research. 2016; 95(13) pp 1452–1456

136. Taddei S, Virdis A, Ghiadoni L, Versari D, Salvetti A. Endothelium, aging, and hypertension. Current Hypertension Reports. 2006; 8(1) pp 84–89

137. Sweazea KL, Johnston CS, Miller B, Gumpricht E. Nitrate-Rich Fruit and Vegetable Supplement Reduces Blood Pressure in Normotensive Healthy Young Males without Significantly Altering Flow-Mediated Vasodilation: A Randomized, Double-Blinded, Controlled Trial. Journal of Nutrition and Metabolism. 2018. 1729653

138. Kapil V, Khambata RS, Robertson A, Caulfield MJ, Ahluwalia A. Dietary nitrate provides sustained blood pressure lowering in hypertensive patients: a randomized, phase 2, double-blind, placebo-controlled study. Hypertension. 2015; 65(2) pp 320–327

139. Bahadoran Z, Mirmiran P, Kabir A, Azizi F, Ghasemi A. The Nitrate-Independent Blood Pressure-Lowering Effect of Beetroot

Juice: A Systematic Review and Meta-Analysis [published correction appears in Advances in Nutrition. 2018 May 1; 9(3) 274]. Advances in Nutrition. 2017; 8(6) pp 830–838

140. EUsalt [Internet]. https://eusalt.com/

141. The Salt Institute to dissolve [Internet]. Food Business News. 2019 https://www.foodbusinessnews.net/articles/13448-the-salt-institute-to-dissolve

142. Mente A, O'Donnell M, Rangarajan S, McQueen M, Dagenais G, Wielgosz A, Lear S, Ah ST, Wei L, Diaz R, Avezum A. Urinary sodium excretion, blood pressure, cardiovascular disease, and mortality: a community-level prospective epidemiological cohort study. The Lancet. 2018; 392(10146) pp 496–506

143. Subway Nutrition Information [Internet]. Subway. 2021 https://www.subway.com/-/media/New_Zealand/Documents/Nutritionals/NZ-Nutritional-Summary.pdf

144. Salt reduction [Internet]. World Health Organization. 2020 https://www.who.int/news-room/fact-sheets/detail/salt-reduction

145. Shaking the Salt Habit to Lower High Blood Pressure [Internet]. Heart. 2016 https://www.heart.org/en/health-topics/high-blood-pressure/changes-you-can-make-to-manage-high-blood-pressure/shaking-the-salt-habit-to-lower-high-blood-pressure

146. Huang L, Trieu K, Yoshimura S, Neal B, Woodward M, Campbell NR, Li Q, Lackland DT, Leung AA, Anderson CA, MacGregor GA. Effect of dose and duration of reduction in dietary sodium on blood pressure levels: systematic review and meta-analysis of randomised trials. BMJ 2020; 368

147. Jones DW, Luft FC, Whelton PK, Alderman MH, Hall JE, Peterson ED, Califf RM, McCarron DA. Can We End the Salt Wars With a Randomized Clinical Trial in a Controlled Environment? Hypertension. 2018; 72(1) pp 10–11

148. Action on Salt [Internet]. http://www.actiononsalt.org.uk/

149. McKay DL, Chen CO, Saltzman E, Blumberg JB. Hibiscus sabdariffa L. tea (tisane) lowers blood pressure in prehypertensive and mildly hypertensive adults. The Journal of Nutrition. 2010; 140(2) pp 298–303

150. Herrera-Arellano A, Flores-Romero S, Chávez-Soto MA, Tortoriello J. Effectiveness and tolerability of a standardized

extract from Hibiscus sabdariffa in patients with mild to moderate hypertension: a controlled and randomized clinical trial. Phytomedicine. 2004; 11(5) pp 375–382

151. Mozaffari-Khosravi H, Jalali-Khanabadi BA, Afkhami-Ardekani M, Fatehi F, Noori-Shadkam M. The effects of sour tea (Hibiscus sabdariffa) on hypertension in patients with type II diabetes. Journal of Human Hypertension. 2009; 23(1) pp 48–54

152. Hopkins AL, Lamm MG, Funk JL, Ritenbaugh C. Hibiscus sabdariffa L. in the treatment of hypertension and hyperlipidemia: a comprehensive review of animal and human studies. Fitoterapia. 2013; 85 pp 84–94

153. Ghayur MN, Gilani AH. Ginger lowers blood pressure through blockade of voltage-dependent calcium channels. Journal of Cardiovascular Pharmacology. 2005; 45(1) pp 74–80

154. Wang Y, Yu H, Zhang X, Feng Q, Guo X, Li S, Li R, Chu D, Ma Y. Evaluation of daily ginger consumption for the prevention of chronic diseases in adults: A cross-sectional study. Nutrition. 2017; 36 pp 79–84

155. Hasani H, Arab A, Hadi A, Pourmasoumi M, Ghavami A, Miraghajani M. Does ginger supplementation lower blood pressure? A systematic review and meta-analysis of clinical trials. Phytotherapy Research. 2019; 33(6) pp 1639–1640

156. Verma SK, Jain V, Katewa SS. Blood pressure lowering, fibrinolysis enhancing and antioxidant activities of cardamom (Elettaria cardamomum). Indian Journal of Biochemistry and Biophysics. 2009; 46 pp 503–506

157. Luo C, Zou L, Sun H, Peng J, Gao C, Bao L, Ji R, Jin Y, Sun S. A Review of the Anti-Inflammatory Effects of Rosmarinic Acid on Inflammatory Diseases. Frontiers in Pharmacology. 2020; 11 pp 153

158. Li QL, Li BG, Zhang Y, Gao XP, Li CQ, Zhang GL. Three angiotensin-converting enzyme inhibitors from Rabdosia coetsa. Phytomedicine. 2008; 15(5) pp 386–388

159. Ferreira LG, Evora PR, Capellini VK, Albuquerque AA, Carvalho MT, da Silva Gomes RA, Parolini MT, Celotto AC. Effect of rosmarinic acid on the arterial blood pressure in normotensive

and hypertensive rats: Role of ACE. Phytomedicine. 2018; 38 pp 158–165

160. Ajebli M, Eddouks M. Antihypertensive activity of Petroselinum crispum through inhibition of vascular calcium channels in rats. Journal of Ethnopharmacology. 2019; 242 pp 112039

161. Umar A, Imam G, Yimin W, Kerim P, Tohti I, Berké B, Moore N. Antihypertensive effects of Ocimum basilicum L. (OBL) on blood pressure in renovascular hypertensive rats. Hypertension Research. 2010; 33(7) pp 727–730

162. Amrani S, Harnafi H, Gadi D, Mekhfi H, Legssyer A, Aziz M, Martin-Nizard F, Bosca L. Vasorelaxant and anti-platelet aggregation effects of aqueous Ocimum basilicum extract. Journal of Ethnopharmacology. 2009; 125(1) pp 157–162

163. Tohti I, Tursun M, Umar A, Turdi S, Imin H, Moore N. Aqueous extracts of Ocimum basilicum L. (sweet basil) decrease platelet aggregation induced by ADP and thrombin in vitro and rats arterio-venous shunt thrombosis in vivo. Thrombosis Research. 2006; 118(6) pp 157–162

164. Peixoto-Neves D, Leal-Cardoso JH, Jaggar JH. Eugenol dilates rat cerebral arteries by inhibiting smooth muscle cell voltage-dependent calcium channels. Journal of Cardiovascular Pharmacology. 2014; 64(5) pp 401–406

165. Kuramochi T, Chu J, Suga T. Gou-teng (from Uncaria rhynchophylla Miquel)-induced endothelium-dependent and -independent relaxations in the isolated rat aorta. Life Sciences. 1994; 54(26) pp 2061–2069

166. Yuzurihara M, Ikarashi Y, Goto K, Sakakibara I, Hayakawa T, Sasaki H. Geissoschizine methyl ether, an indole alkaloid extracted from Uncariae Ramulus et Uncus, is a potent vasorelaxant of isolated rat aorta. European Journal of Pharmacology. 2002; 444(3) pp 183–189

167. Schüssler M, Hölzl J, Fricke U. Myocardial effects of flavonoids from Crataegus species. Arzneimittel-forschung. 1995; 45(8) pp 842–845

168. Brixius K, Willms S, Napp A, Tossios P, Ladage D, Bloch W, Mehlhorn U, Schwinger RH. Crataegus special extract WS 1442 induces an endothelium-dependent, NO-mediated

vasorelaxation via eNOS-phosphorylation at serine 1177. Cardiovascular Drugs and Therapy. 2006; 20(3) pp 177–184

169. Zhu J, Zhang Y, Yang C. Protective effect of 3-n-butylphthalide against hypertensive nephropathy in spontaneously hypertensive rats. Molecular Medicine Reports. 2014; 11(2) pp 1448–1454

170. Madhavi D, Kagan D, Rao V. A Pilot Study to Evaluate the Antihypertensive Effect of a Celery Extract in Mild to Moderate Hypertensive Patients. Natural Medicine Journal. 2013; 4(4) pp 185–189

171. Tashakori-Sabzevar F, Razavi BM, Imenshahidi M, Daneshmandi M, Fatehi H, Sarkarizi YE, Mohajeri SA. Evaluation of mechanism for antihypertensive and vasorelaxant effects of hexanic and hydroalcoholic extracts of celery seed in normotensive and hypertensive rats. Revista Brasileira de Farmacognosia. 2016; 5 pp 619–626

172. Matic I, Guidi A, Kenzo M, Mattei M, Galgani A. Investigation of medicinal plants traditionally used as dietary supplements: A review on Moringa oleifera. Journal of Public Health in Africa. 2018; 9(3) pp 841

173. Mahomoodally MF. Traditional medicines in Africa: an appraisal of ten potent African medicinal plants. Evidence-Based Complementary and Alternative Medicine. 2013 617459

174. Randriamboavonjy JI, Loirand G, Vaillant N, Lauzier B, Derbré S, Michalet S, Pacaud P, Tesse A. Cardiac Protective Effects of Moringa oleifera Seeds in Spontaneous Hypertensive Rats. American Journal of Hypertension. 2016; 29(7) pp 873–881

175. Faizi S, Siddiqui BS, Saleem R, Siddiqui S, Aftab K. Fully acetylated carbamate and hypotensive thiocarbamate glycosides from Moringa oleifera. Phytochemistry. 1995; 38(4) pp 957–963

176. Faizi S, Siddiqui BS, Saleem R, Siddiqui S, Aftab K, Gilani AU. Isolation and structure elucidation of new nitrile and mustard oil glycosides from Moringa oleifera and their effect on blood pressure. Journal of Natural Products. 1994; 57(9) pp 1256–1261

177. Faizi S, Siddiqui BS, Saleem R, Aftab K, Shaheen F. Hypotensive constituents from the pods of Moringa oleifera. Planta Medica. 1998; 64(03) pp 225–228

178. Aekthammarat D, Tangsucharit P, Pannangpetch P, Sriwantana T, Sibmooh N. Moringa oleifera leaf extract enhances endothelial nitric oxide production leading to relaxation of resistance artery and lowering of arterial blood pressure. Biomedicine Pharmacotherapy. 2020; 130 pp 110605

179. Khan H, Jaiswal V, Kulshreshtha S, Khan A. Potential Angiotensin Converting Enzyme Inhibitors from Moringa oleifera. Recent Patents on Biotechnology. 2019; 13(3) pp 239–248

180. Hodgson JM, Puddey IB, Burke V, Beilin LJ, Jordan N. Effects on blood pressure of drinking green and black tea. Journal of Hypertension. 1999; 17(4) pp 457–463

181. Yarmolinsky J, Gon G, Edwards P. Effect of tea on blood pressure for secondary prevention of cardiovascular disease: a systematic review and meta-analysis of randomized controlled trials. Nutrition Reviews. 2015; 73(4) pp 236–246

182. Nogueira LP, Nogueira Neto JF, Klein MR, Sanjuliani AF. Short-term Effects of Green Tea on Blood Pressure, Endothelial Function, and Metabolic Profile in Obese Prehypertensive Women: A Crossover Randomized Clinical Trial. Journal of the American College of Nutrition. 2017; 36(2) pp 108–115

183. Hurst WJ, Krake SH, Bergmeier SC, Payne MJ, Miller KB, Stuart DA. Impact of fermentation, drying, roasting and Dutch processing on flavan-3-ol stereochemistry in cacao beans and cocoa ingredients. Chemistry Central Journal. 2011; 5(1) pp 53

184. Jalil AM, Ismail A. Polyphenols in cocoa and cocoa products: is there a link between antioxidant properties and health? Molecules. 2008; 13(9) pp 2190–2219

185. Hollenberg NK, Fisher ND, McCullough ML. Flavanols, the Kuna, cocoa consumption, and nitric oxide. Journal of the American Society of Hypertension. 2009; 3(2) pp 105–112

186. Buijsse B, Feskens EJ, Kok FJ, Kromhout D. Cocoa intake, blood pressure, and cardiovascular mortality: the Zutphen Elderly Study. Archives of Internal Medicine. 2006; 166(4) pp 411–417

187. Faridi Z, Njike VY, Dutta S, Ali A, Katz DL. Acute dark chocolate and cocoa ingestion and endothelial function: a randomized controlled crossover trial. The American Journal of Clinical Nutrition. 2008; 88(1) pp 58–63

188. Grassi D, Desideri G, Necozione S, Lippi C, Casale R, Properzi G, Blumberg JB, Ferri C. Blood pressure is reduced and insulin sensitivity increased in glucose-intolerant, hypertensive subjects after 15 days of consuming high-polyphenol dark chocolate. The Journal of Nutrition. 2008; 138(9) pp 1671–1676

189. Grassi D, Necozione S, Lippi C, Croce G, Valeri L, Pasqualetti P, Desideri G, Blumberg JB, Ferri C. Cocoa reduces blood pressure and insulin resistance and improves endothelium-dependent vasodilation in hypertensives. Hypertension. 2005; 46(2) pp 398–405

190. Fisher ND, Hughes M, Gerhard-Herman M, Hollenberg NK. Flavanol-rich cocoa induces nitric-oxide-dependent vasodilation in healthy humans. Journal of Hypertension. 2003; 21(12) pp 2281–2286

191. Franco R, Oñatibia-Astibia A, Martínez-Pinilla E. Health benefits of methylxanthines in cacao and chocolate. Nutrients. 2013; 5(10) pp 4159–4173

192. Allicin [Internet]. Wikipedia. 2020 https://en.wikipedia.org/wiki/Allicin

193. Song K, Milner JA. The Influence of Heating on the Anticancer Properties of Garlic. The Journal of Nutrition. 2001; 121(3) pp 1054S–1057S

194. Piano MR, Burke L, Kang M, Phillips SA. Effects of Repeated Binge Drinking on Blood Pressure Levels and Other Cardiovascular Health Metrics in Young Adults: National Health and Nutrition Examination Survey, 2011-2014. Journal of the American Heart Association. 2018; 7(13) e008733

195. Klatsky AL, Friedman GD, Siegelaub AB, Gérard MJ. Alcohol Consumption and Blood Pressure: Kaiser-Permanente Multiphasic Health Examination Data. New England Journal of Medicine. 1977; 296(21) pp 1194–1200

196. Roerecke M, Kaczorowski J, Tobe SW, Gmel G, Hasan OS, Rehm J. The effect of a reduction in alcohol consumption on blood pressure: a systematic review and meta-analysis. The Lancet Publish Health. 2017; 2(2) pp e108–e120

197. What is a standard drink? [Internet]. NIAAA https://www.niaaa.nih.gov/alcohols-effects-health/overview-alcohol-consumption/what-standard-drink

198. Grassi GM, Somers VK, Renk WS, Abboud FM, Mark AL. Effects of alcohol intake on blood pressure and sympathetic nerve activity in normotensive humans: a preliminary report. Official Journal of the International Society of Hypertension. 1989; 7(6) pp S20–S21

199. Schrieks IC, Stafleu A, Kallen VL, Grootjen M, Witkamp RF, Hendriks HF. Moderate alcohol consumption, autonomic nervous system and mood. Appetite. 2013; 71 pp 485

200. Cushman WC. Alcohol Consumption and Hypertension. The Journal of Clinical Hypertension. 2007; 3(3) pp 166–170

201. Can Alcohol Cause High Blood Pressure (Alcohol and Blood Pressure) [Internet]. The Dr Joe. 2019 https://thedrjoe.com/can-alcohol-cause-high-blood-pressure

202. Telles S, Verma S, Sharma SK, Gupta RK, Balkrishna A. Alternate-nostril yoga breathing reduced blood pressure while increasing performance in a vigilance test. Medical Science Monitor Basic Research. 2017; 23 pp 392–398

203. Chen YF, Huang XY, Chien CH, Cheng JF. The effectiveness of diaphragmatic breathing relaxation training for reducing anxiety. Perspectives in Psychiatric Care. 2017; 53(4) pp 329–336

204. 22 Facts About the Brain [Internet]. DENT Neurological Institute. 2019 https://www.dentinstitute.com/posts/lifestyle-tips/22-facts-about-the-brain-world-brain-day/

205. Archer SN, Robilliard DL, Skene DJ, Smits M, Williams A, Arendt J, von Schantz M. A length polymorphism in the circadian clock gene PER3 is linked to delayed sleep phase syndrome and extreme diurnal preference. Sleep. 2003; 26(4) pp 413–415

206. Samson DR, Crittenden AN, Mabulla IA, Mabulla AZ, Nunn CL. Chronotype variation drives night-time sentinel-like behaviour in hunter-gatherers. Proceedings of the Royal Society B: Biological Sciences. 2017; 284(1858) pp 20170967

207. Rutters F, Lemmens SG, Adam TC, Bremmer MA, Elders PJ, Nijpels G, Dekker JM. Is social jetlag associated with an adverse endocrine, behavioral, and cardiovascular risk profile? Journal of Biological Rhythms. 2014; 29(5) pp 377–383

208. Physical Activity to Prevent and Treat Hypertension: A Systematic Review [Internet]. Research Gate. 2019 https://www.researchgate.

net/profile/Linda-Pescatello/publication/333535814_Physical_
Activity_to_Prevent_and_Treat_Hypertension_A_Systematic_
Review/links/5fd7902d92851c13fe86f1f2/Physical-Activity-to-
Prevent-and-Treat-Hypertension-A-Systematic-Review.pdf

209. Brook RD, Appel LJ, Rubenfire M, Ogedegbe G, Bisognano JD, Elliott WJ, Fuchs FD, Hughes JW, Lackland DT, Staffileno BA, Townsend RR. American Heart Association Professional Education Committee of the Council for High Blood Pressure Research, Council on Cardiovascular and Stroke Nursing, Council on Epidemiology and Prevention, and Council on Nutrition, Physical Activity. Beyond medications and diet: alternative approaches to lowering blood pressure: a scientific statement from the American Heart Association. Hypertension. 2016; 61(6) pp 1360–1383

210. Piepoli MF, Abreu A, Albus C, Ambrosetti M, Brotons C, Catapano AL, Corra U, Cosyns B, Deaton C, Graham I, Hoes A. Update on cardiovascular prevention in clinical practice: a position paper of the European Association of Preventive Cardiology of the European Society of Cardiology. European Journal of Preventative Cardiology. 2020; 27(2) pp 181–205

211. Pescatello LS, Buchner DM, Jakicic JM, Powell KE, Kraus WE, Bloodgood B, Campbell WW, Dietz S, DiPietro L, George SM, Macko RF. Physical activity to prevent and treat hypertension: a systematic review. Medicine & Science in Sports & Exercise. 2019; 51(6) pp 1314–1323

212. Hanssen H, Boardman H, Deiseroth A, Moholdt T, Simonenko M, Kränkel N, Niebauer J, Tiberi M, Abreu A, Solberg EE, Pescatello L. Personalized exercise prescription in the prevention and treatment of arterial hypertension: a Consensus Document from the European Association of Preventive Cardiology (EAPC) and the ESC Council on Hypertension. European Journal of Preventive Cardiology. 2022; 29(1) pp 205–215

213. Cramer H, Sellin C, Schumann D, Dobos G. Yoga in Arterial Hypertension: A Three-Armed, Randomized Controlled Trial. Deutsches Ärzteblatt International. 2018; 115(50) pp 833–839

214. Cramer H. The Efficacy and Safety of Yoga in Managing Hypertension. Experimental and Clinical Endocrinology & Diabetes. 2016; 124(02) pp 65–70

Printed in Great Britain
by Amazon

44565759R00195